VEGAN
MASTER PLAN

How to Become Healthier, Happier, and Stronger on the Vegan Diet

ANNETTE SHAW

NEWMAN SPRINGS PUBLISHING
Meadville, PA

First originally published by Newman Springs Publishing 2025

ISBN 978-1-64096-028-2 (Paperback)
ISBN 978-1-64096-032-9 (Digital)

Printed in the United States of America

Vegan Master Plan

THIS DOCUMENT IS geared toward providing exact and reliable information with regards to the topic and issue covered. The publication is sold with the idea that the publisher is not required to render accounting, officially permitted or otherwise, qualified services. If advice is necessary, legal or professional, a practiced individual in the profession should be ordered from a declaration of principles, which was accepted and approved equally by a Committee of the American Bar Association and a Committee of Publishers and Associations.

In no way is it legal to reproduce, duplicate or transmit any part of this document by either electronic means or in printed format. Recording of this publication is strictly prohibited, and any storage of this document is not allowed unless with written permission from the publisher. All rights reserved.

The information provided herein is stated to be truthful and consistent, in that any liability in terms of inattention or otherwise, by any usage or abuse of any policies, processes or directions contained within is the solitary and utter responsibility of the recipient reader. Under no circumstances will any legal responsibility or blame be held against the publisher for any reparation, damages, or monetary loss due to the information herein, either directly or indirectly.

Respective authors own all copyrights not held by the publisher.

The information herein is offered solely for informational purposes and is universal as so. The presentation of the information is without contract or any type of guarantee assurance.

The trademarks that are used are without any consent, and the publication of the trademark is without permission or backing by the trademark owner. All trademarks and brands within this book are for clarifying purposes only and are owned by the owners themselves, not affiliated with this document.

Contents

Introduction

ARE YOU THINKING about taking the plunge and becoming a vegan, but you don't have a clue where to start? Perhaps you've just seen one of the many documentaries highlighting the cruelty of the meat industry and have vowed to change your own life and save the lives of hundreds of animals in the process. Maybe your kids have just started asking, "Where does our meat come from, Mommy?" and they don't mean from the local supermarket. You get that uneasy sick feeling in the pit of your stomach, knowing the horrendous truths that lie behind the meat industry. Or maybe you're just sick of feeling unhealthy and tired all the time and think that your malaise might have something to do with your diet.

Whatever your reason, you've come to the right place.

I've been where you are right now, and I understand how confusing it can be, not knowing where to start or exactly what to do. Luckily, I can give you a firsthand account of what wonders await you when you start adopting a healthy vegan lifestyle, as well as what horrors happen within your body when you don't (or can't) educate yourself about the vegan diet. Most importantly, with this book, you'll learn about optimal meat-free nutrition.

This is my guide to veganism. I share with you my knowledge on how to properly enjoy the incredible benefits of this environmentally friendly lifestyle without compromising your health.

In this guide, you'll discover everything you need to know to get started on a healthy, cruelty-free, and environmentally friendly diet and learn everything you need to take that all-important first step that will change your life forever. Most importantly, you'll find out about the key facts about good nutrition that will get your skin glowing, your hair and eyes shining with health, and your entire body overflowing with brand-new plant-based energy.

There are several ways you can read this book. You can read my every word from cover to cover, or you can dip in and out and select the nuggets of information that will really make a difference to you and your life. I don't mind—it's for you to decide.

Before you get started, though, let me share with you my story of how, years ago, I ended up making a major decision that would change my life for the better.

I'll never forget the precise moment when I vowed never to let meat pass my lips again.

It was a bright day in April, and I was frying fish in my kitchen at home, singing along to my favorite song and enjoying all the hope that a little sunshine can bring. Spring was in the air, and I was feeling so good! I slid the cooked fish from the skillet onto my plate, went to grab some cutlery, and sat down in my usual place at the table, still humming happily to myself. I raised my fork ready to tuck in when I noticed something. That silver fish lay wide-eyed on my plate, and all I could see was death staring back up at me. Death and suffering. I couldn't shake the feeling.

I had to look away to avoid its accusing stare. I pushed the plate away in disgust and turned my attention to emptying the contents of my fridge. Never again would I eat another living creature. Ever.

This wasn't the first time I'd seen a shift in my perception about my food choices. Several months earlier, the blood dripping from frying hamburger had caught my eye, and I instantly connected this seemingly inert food stuff to the living, breathing, and feeling creatures that we share the world with. Then, a few weeks later, the whole process of grilling chicken legs at a company cookout turned my stomach, and I just couldn't do it anymore. I just couldn't eat meat.

Like many others, I'd realized that eating meat causes intense suffering for countless innocent animals. I also realized that the vegan lifestyle was a much healthier choice for humans. So from that point onward, I vowed to make more spiritual, more humane, and healthier food choices in the future.

So can you.

You might not be fully aware of the grim realities of the meat industry yet, and that's okay. They don't want you to know. They don't want you to comprehend the terrible conditions and the horrendous sights and smells. They don't want you to find out about the extent of the suffering each animal that lands on dinner plates has gone through. They just want your dollars.

I, on the other hand, want you to know the truth. I want to tell you about my story and want to share with you the wonders I've experienced since going vegan. This is the story of how I became a vegan and how I remain one to this very day. This is a collection of all the important bits that I've gathered along the way that I feel would be helpful to others.

Everyone has their very own path to tread on the way to kinder, healthier, and more spiritual eating. Over sixteen million people in the United States alone conform to a vegan diet. Behind that are sixteen million different reasons and situations that have led people to make a choice that would change their lives for the better. Whatever your reason may be, allow me to offer a lending hand or perhaps a guiding voice in your journey to health and fulfillment. We may all have our own paths to tread, but together, we can make each other's journey happier, easier, and ultimately, more rewarding.

Part I

All About Veganism

In this part, we'll discuss the basics of what veganism really is. We'll talk about all the different diets or lifestyles that fall under the general term that is veganism, as well as correct any common misconceptions you might have about this amazing yet often misunderstood lifestyle.

Chapter 1

What Is Veganism?

So, FIRST THINGS first, what exactly is veganism?

When people say veganism, most will probably just think about a meatless diet. There is much, much more to veganism than just no-meat, however. For me, veganism isn't just a diet. It's a lifestyle. It's about making a commitment to providing your body with the proper nourishment it needs and deserves. It's also about adopting changes in the way you live your life that go against unethical practices that harm innocent animals and slowly destroy the world we live in. It's about thinking of your overall well-being and becoming one with nature.

Below, we'll discuss the different facets of vegetarianism vs veganism that you might encounter along the way.

The Different Types of Vegetarians vs Vegans

In truth, vegetarianism is simply a catchall term for the many different types of lifestyles that fall under the same general group. Just as people come in many different shapes, colors, and sizes, vegetarians too are quite varied and diverse, and each has their own approach to living as a vegetarian. Here are some of the general categories that vegetarians fall under:

3

- *Lacto-ovo vegetarians* are vegetarians who avoid meat, fish, poultry, and seafood. Lacto-ovo vegetarians are also known as true vegetarians, since they are the most common kind, and they are also what most people imagine when they hear the term *vegetarian.*
- *Lacto-vegetarians*, meanwhile, are vegetarians who not only avoid meat, fish, poultry, and seafood but also stay away from eggs too. They do, however, consume other forms of dairy, such as milk and cheese.
- *Ovo-vegetarians*, on the other hand, avoid meat, fish, poultry, seafood, and dairy, but they are fine with consuming eggs.
- *Semivegetarians*, lastly, although not technically vegetarians in the strictest sense, are those who haven't completely eliminated meat from their diet. Semivegetarians may be *pescatarians*, who consume fish and seafood but avoid other animal meat. Or they may be *pollotarians*, who consume poultry but avoid fish, seafood, and other animal meats. Some semivegetarians also predominantly avoid meat, except for just a few times each month.
- *Vegans* take vegetarianism to another level by avoiding things that other vegetarians may consume. They stay away from meat, fish, poultry, seafood, dairy, eggs, and even animal by-products, such as gelatin and honey. Besides that, many vegans also avoid nonfood products that are made from animals, such as leather, wool, or cosmetics.

Now that you're more familiar with what veganism is, let's talk about what veganism *isn't*, or about some of the common misconceptions people have about the vegan lifestyle.

Chapter 2

Common Myths and Misconceptions About Veganism

VEGANISM IS A pretty controversial topic. With the whole world seemingly too keen to share well-meaning, but often misinformed, nuggets of information about this topic, it would be a great help to dispel some of these myths before we can move on to tackling the finer details of veganism and plant-based nutrition. Below are some of the most common myths that are spread about veganism. Let's see how many of these you've heard before!

"Vegans don't get enough protein"

If I ask you to think of sources of protein, what's the first thing that comes to mind? I can pretty much guarantee that you'll have large slabs of meat in your thoughts, and you might fall into the trap of believing that only meat (and, perhaps, fish) is a reliable source of protein. Ditching meat means ditching protein, right? Well, that's where you are wrong.

Luckily for vegans, meat is not the sole source of protein in this world. Nature is kind and has provided abundant amounts of protein in every living thing, whether animal or plant. That means that you really don't need to be too worried about protein when you follow a vegan diet. In fact, many common vegetables contain a lot more protein than you need. Theoretically, you could eat soybeans for the rest of your life and still get enough protein in your diet!

"Vegan life is tough, since you have to live only on salads"

Yes, living solely on salads would be tough, but there's really no reason to worry, since there is so much more to veganism then eating salad all day! Just ask any gourmet vegan chef.

Vegan life is brimming with a variety of healthy options. Although you can have as much salad as you want, in reality, the sky is the limit in terms of possibilities of vegan choices!

"The human body was designed to eat meat, and veganism is going against what nature intended"

The people who say veganism is against nature couldn't be more wrong. We only need to consider our shiny teeth and lengthy intestines for proof. If we were "designed" to eat meat, then we wouldn't share the same coiling intestines as our herbivore cousins. We wouldn't have teeth designed for grinding and eating veggies and would instead have mouths full of doglike, meat-tearing teeth. Carnivores have short intestines in order to eliminate digested meat before it rots (yuck!), and those tearing teeth are especially meant for munching on their favorite hunks of meat—a far cry from what we as human beings have in our anatomy. Yes, humans are capable of eating meat, but we can also eat vegetables. We are lucky enough to be able to choose, and it's important to choose what is healthy and good for our bodies over what hurts us in the long run.

"Vegans regularly feel deprived because of their diets"

This is another blatantly wrong statement. Why would I feel deprived? It's not like I've drastically limited the amount of food I consume or stopped eating completely. Instead, I've simply opened my mind to all of the wonderful healthy options out there. Becoming vegan has driven me to explore all of the numerous flavorful foods and cuisines available. I would never have had the opportunity to try out some of the most delicious meals I've had in my life had I not become vegan. It's all a matter of perspective, and from the perspective of someone who's been a vegan for decades, I can say that no, I haven't been deprived, and instead, I have gained so much more from choosing to become a vegan.

— Part II —

Making the Switch to Veganism

Now that you've learned about what veganism is and isn't, let's get on to what might just be the most interesting and exciting part for you: making the switch to veganism. Here, you'll learn more about the many different reasons that make the vegan lifestyle as amazing as it is. Besides that, you'll also receive some great tips on how to get started on your vegan journey so that your own switch can become as smooth and easy as possible.

Chapter 3

Why Switch to Veganism?

OF COURSE, THE big question is why should we give up meat and switch to veganism? Well, there is a myriad of compelling health, environmental, ethical, and other reasons to cut meat from your lifestyle. Before we get into all of those reasons in detail, however, let's examine the place that meat holds in our lives today to gain a better understanding of how important it is to make the smart choice and go vegan.

The Meat Tradition

It is undeniable that meat has become an integral part of the way we celebrate many important events in our lives.

In a way, meat has become synonymous with celebrations. Think about it. When we say Thanksgiving, often, the first thing that comes to mind is the turkey. At Easter, meanwhile, ham often takes center stage as the traditional meal. Then, when summer comes around, countless hungry mouths often wait for the first burger patties or steaks to hit the grill.

However, we as a species were probably meant to eat vegetables, fruits, nuts, berries, and legumes. The structure of our jaws, the shape of our teeth, the muscles in our faces, and the saliva in our mouths all share more similarities with herbivorous animals than carnivores.

If we were meant to eat plants, how then did we manage to end up treating meat as a central part of many of our celebrations?

Well, we can imagine that eating meat was initially an opportunistic event, born of the need to survive. When early groups of men moved to a hunter-gatherer orientation, it made sense that they turned to meat, considering the availability of resources, the taste of cooked meat, and the sustained energy received from the high-fat content in meat. It was in these circumstances where meat might have found its roots as an integral part of communal celebrations.

In those days, for instance, finding cooked meat from, say, a forest fire, would have been a cause for celebration, and partaking in that fortunate bounty would have been something that entire clans would have participated in. Back then, meat was an important piece in the larger picture of community life. Hunting, for example, was often a group effort, with teams working together to track, hunt down, and finally kill their prey. Entire clans relied on the success of these hunts, and bringing home the carcass of a slain animal would have meant food not just for the individual, but for the numerous other clan members who relied on the hunters for sustenance. Thus, for those who waited for the return of the hunters, the sight of meat would most definitely have been greeted with cheers, as it meant that they could fill their stomachs for yet another day. In addition, once the animal was brought back to the clan, it would also have taken a group effort to skin the animal and tear or cut the meat from the carcass. Everyone would have participated in this and subsequently shared in the rewards of their work. It's easy to see, then, how meat could have become central in the need for gathering and celebration so deeply ingrained in our collective cultures. We celebrate the different seasons and the multitude of life events with family and friends, and because many celebrations for early humans involved eating meat, that tradition has continued in modern times.

The problem, however, is that food should nourish and feed the body and leave us energized and refreshed. The human body is a machine that needs the right fuel to keep it running in peak condition. When our bodies suffer from high blood pressure, type 2 diabetes, or high cholesterol, they are essentially like car engines that haven't been tuned or aren't running on the optimal type of fuel they need to run efficiently. As with cars, our bodies need the right kind of fuel to run at peak efficiency. And high-fat meat and meat that's been fed antibiotics throughout its life are simply not the kind of fuel the human body was meant to run on. Fortunately, the vegan diet is available to fuel your body the proper way. So if eating unhealthy meat is like loading up your shiny sports car with diesel fuel that is inappropriate and damaging to its engine, then eating vegan is just like filling up your tank with the best high-grade car gasoline that money can buy.

Now that we know why meat isn't the right food for our bodies, let's talk about some of the most compelling reasons to make the switch to veganism, starting with health.

Health Reasons

Simply put, following a proper vegan diet is miles away the healthier choice. Countless scientific studies and personal experiences have shown just how amazing a vegan lifestyle can be for our bodies.

Diseases

In terms of diseases, veganism can go a very long way in ensuring that our bodies stay disease-free. Adopting a plant-based diet can have many beneficial effects on your overall health, and in this section, we'll discuss how veganism can help address many of the problems related to some of the most common medical conditions among humans today.

Heart Disease

Studies show that vegans experience lower levels of cholesterol, are less likely to have trouble managing their blood pressure, and enjoy a significantly lower risk for heart disease, type 2 diabetes, and stroke.

Vegan diets are low in saturated fat. Saturated fat primarily comes from meat and can be transformed into cholesterol. Cholesterol, in turn, lines the arteries and impedes the flow of blood, leading to heart disease and strokes. Vegan diets avoid this problem entirely, as they contain virtually no cholesterol at all.

While you do need to consume some fat to stay healthy, vegans still have the upper hand, as they use the healthy kind of fat—unsaturated fat—found in plant oils, such as coconut oil and olive oil, most of which are taken from seeds.

Furthermore, vegan diets are also high in soluble fiber, which is typically found in vegetables, whole grains, and beans, among other items. Soluble fiber absorbs a lot of the nasty cholesterol that ends up hurting our bodies, providing yet another reason for vegans to be healthy and happy.

Last, plants contain chemicals that help our hearts out. Many fruits and vegetables contain phytosterols and other antioxidants, which fight heart disease. The bottom line is if you want to keep your heart beating healthily for years to come, veganism is the way to go!

Hypertension

Somewhat related to heart disease, hypertension is otherwise known as the condition of having high blood pressure. Hypertension is very common among meat-eating populations and comes with symptoms such as headaches, fatigue, dizziness, and a general ill feeling. Not just that, having elevated blood pressure levels could also lead to a heart attack or stroke.

Of course, a vegan diet can do wonders countering hypertension. First, vegan diets can help with weight loss due to the lower calorie count of vegan foods. This is great news for those who struggle with high blood pressure, as hypertension is strongly linked with being overweight. As your weight drops, so too should your blood pressure, leaving you feeling not just lighter, but better, overall!

Second, sodium chloride, or the table salt that most people use in just about every meal, can also contribute to high blood pressure. When we consume too much salt, that salt ends up in the bloodstream, making it more difficult for the kidneys to filter our blood. As a result, more water ends up in the bloodstream to balance out the salt content, thus increasing our blood pressure. Thankfully, most vegan foods naturally come without salt (unless of course, we add salt to the dishes ourselves), giving hypertension sufferers another way to naturally lower their blood pressure levels!

Last, many plant-based foods are high in minerals, such as potassium and magnesium, which help combat high blood pressure. Many of these plant-based foods form a large part of vegan diets, meaning you could already be lowering your blood pressure without even giving much thought to it, simply by going vegan!

Type 2 Diabetes

In part because of the large quantity of unhealthy food that we, as a species, have grown used to consuming, millions of people around the world now suffer from diabetes. In fact, obesity and the high consumption of sugar and unsaturated fats have both been linked with an increased risk for type 2 diabetes. While sweet sugary foods may be an amazing treat for most people, shoveling down too much of them can be like dumping sugar straight into our bloodstreams, forcing our pancreases to work harder to produce insulin. The bodies of people with type 2 diabetes form what is called an insulin resistance, which means that their cells do not respond normally to the insulin that should be regulating blood glucose levels. As a result, blood glucose levels remain elevated for extended periods of time. In the long run, type 2 diabetes can cause cell damage, loss of eyesight, kidney problems, loss of limbs, impeded digestion, nerve damage, and a host of other medical complications.

Living a healthy vegan lifestyle can go a long way in fighting the type 2 diabetes that plagues so many people around the world today. Vegan diets typically tend to come with large amounts of complex carbohydrates. Complex carbohydrates have a low glycemic index, and foods with a low glycemic index contain the fiber that our bodies need to help deal with the simple sugars in our blood.

Cancer

Research from around the world has shown that vegan diets—naturally low in saturated fat, high in fiber, and replete with cancer-protective phytochemicals—help to prevent cancer. Major studies in England and Germany, for example, have shown that vegans are about 40 percent less likely to develop cancer compared to meat-eaters. In the United States, studies of Seventh Day Adventists, who, for religious reasons, are largely lacto-ovo vegetarians, have shown significant reductions in cancer risk among those who avoid meat. Similarly, breast cancer rates have also been shown to be dramatically lower in nations such as China, where plant-based diets are more common. In contrast, in Japan, women who follow Western-style, meat-based diets are eight times more likely to develop breast cancer than women who follow a more traditional plant-based diet. A separate study from Cambridge University, meanwhile, has linked diets high in saturated fat to breast cancer, while another study linked dairy products to an increased risk of ovarian cancer, with the process of breaking down the lactose (milk sugar) evidently being damaging to the ovaries.

It's amazing, isn't it? The difference in the cancer risk for meat-eaters and vegans is as clear as night and day. But how is this so? Well, the simple answer is that vegans, thanks to their diets, naturally stay away from all of the nasty cancer-causing stuff, while, at the same time, consuming more of the things that help keep cancer away.

Vegans avoid the animal fat linked to cancer, and they consume abundant fiber, vitamins, and phytochemicals that help to prevent cancer. Some types of cancer, such as colon and breast cancer, have been linked to obesity, a condition which a vegan lifestyle also helps to fight. Many foods in vegan diets are also packed with antioxidants, which help fight cancer by neutralizing the oxygen free radicals in our bodies that damage our cells and DNA, eventually leading to the onset of the dreaded disease. In addition, blood analysis of vegans reveals a higher level of "natural killer cells," or specialized white blood cells that attack cancer cells.

While it is true that cancer is virtually unpredictable and can strike at any time, adopting a healthy vegan lifestyle is definitely one of the best things you can do to improve your chances and reduce your cancer risk!

Kidney Stones

Kidney stones, otherwise known as renal calculus or nephrolithiasis, is the condition of having solid material, or stones, forming within the kidneys. Kidney stones usually leave the body naturally by passing out with the urine. However, those who have had the condition before know that passing kidney stones through the urine stream can be quite an excruciatingly painful experience, and, as such, it is best to take steps to prevent the stones from forming in the first place.

Diets that are high in protein, especially animal protein, tend to cause the body to excrete more calcium, oxalate, and uric acid. These three substances are the main components of urinary tract stones. British researchers have advised that people with a tendency to form kidney stones should follow a vegan diet. The American Academy of Family Physicians (AAFP) notes that high animal protein intake is largely responsible for the high prevalence of kidney stones in the United States. In addition, physicians in other developed countries recommend protein restriction for the prevention of recurrent kidney stones.

Osteoporosis

Osteoporosis is the leading cause for broken bones in the elderly. Osteoporosis is a disease that weakens bones and makes them more brittle, thus increasing the risk of bone breakage. The trouble with osteoporosis is that it is hard to detect and often has no symptoms. Often, a broken bone is the first sign of the disease. It is indeed quite concerning, but, thankfully, the risk for osteoporosis can be reduced by adhering to a vegan lifestyle. Since animal products force calcium out of the body, eating meat can promote bone loss. In, fact, in nations with mainly vegetable-based diets (and without dairy product consumption), osteoporosis is less common than in the United States, even when the calcium intake in those nations is lower than in the United States.

Many of us continue to consume meat, while at the same time downing calcium supplements and prescription drugs to stave off the disease. The problem, however, is that these drugs can have drastic side effects. Furthermore, most experts agree that calcium supplements are inferior to calcium derived from natural food sources. Doesn't it make more sense (and cents) to get your calcium from eating a healthier plant-based diet?

Tinnitus

It might be surprising to find tinnitus on this list, especially since most physicians and experts will tell you that there is no cure for it, and that those who suffer from it should just learn to live with it as best they can. Tinnitus refers to a constant and annoying ringing in the ears. Based on my personal experience, however, the answer to the question of whether or not tinnitus can be beaten is a resounding *yes*, and I can attest that a healthy vegan lifestyle can play a key role in that recovery.

In simple terms, tinnitus is just like that sound that lingers in your ears after spending a night at a rock concert or a loud nightclub, except it stays on for weeks, months, or even years. This sound may differ, but it is often described as ringing, humming, hissing, buzzing, grinding, or whistling. It might not sound like much of an issue to most people, but as a former tinnitus sufferer myself, I know firsthand how torturous it can be. Focusing in meetings, or even on simpler tasks, can be the most monumental struggle with a constant, never-ending sound in the back of one's head. For some, sleep can become close to impossible. This chronic problem affects the physical and mental well-being of the sufferer and can cause severe additional stress, leading to an overall drop in quality of life, with some people slipping into depression or even contemplating suicide.

To get a better idea of how tinnitus can be beaten, let us first look at how it occurs. The process of hearing begins when the outer ear captures sound waves traveling through the air. The sound waves then reach the eardrum, causing it to vibrate. The vibrations then travel to the three small bones in the inner ear, and then into the cochlea, where the vibrations are converted into nerve signals, and then sent to the brain to process and make sense of. When a person has tinnitus, their nerve cells keep firing away, even in the absence of a sound source. For most people, this is due to a hearing loss, for which the brain tries to compensate, thus causing the symptoms of tinnitus. Other possible causes, however, include head injuries, problems with the inner ear, illness, substance abuse, and long-term chronic stress.

Whatever the cause may be, I have found that beating tinnitus is possible through a multistep process that can be simplified to eliminating the physical causes first, and then making a major positive lifestyle shift. Once you've had your tinnitus diagnosed and have a better clue of its root cause, do what you can to eliminate that cause through medication, surgery, or other treatments. In some lucky cases, tinnitus resolves itself after the root cause has been eliminated. If it doesn't go away, however, most doctors will probably just tell you to give it time, wait, and simply hope for the best, as there isn't much else that can be done.

But there *is* something you can do actually, and this is where the vegan diet comes in. Many people today mistakenly view "health" as simply the absence of disease. In reality, however, there is so much more to health, as it involves the physical, mental, and spiritual well-being of a person. A symptom such as tinnitus can be viewed as sign or consequences of not being in optimal health. By living as healthy of a lifestyle as we can, we minimize the risk for such symptoms.

Living a healthy lifestyle, however, doesn't just help us avoid symptoms. Rather, just as important, it helps our bodies heal and recover as well. Think about it. How can a body weighed down by ill nutrition and high-stress possibly ever effectively and efficiently recover from a symptom? Within the setting of an unhealthy lifestyle, the body simply can't use its resources as best as it can to heal itself because, quite simply, it is too busy working trying to stay afloat.

When we make a major positive shift in the way we treat our bodies, we set the stage and give our bodies the tools they need to do their magic and let healing take its course. Of course, as you probably already know by now, switching to a vegan lifestyle is simply one of the best, most surefire ways of getting there. When we give our bodies the proper nutrition that they need, and on top of that, reduce stress as well, our bodies can do amazing things, and as my own experiences prove, one of those things is beating the maddening and torturous condition known as tinnitus.

Follow the steps outlined in this plan and you will beat that tinnitus.

Optimum Nutrition

Food is vital to human health, so why do we often neglect to pay close enough attention to what we are putting into our bodies? We stuff ourselves with white carbs, processed foods, additives and preservatives, high levels of sugar, fat and thousands of suspect chemicals without a moment's thought as to what it is doing to our bodies.

But this needs to stop right here, right now. We can't continue to gorge ourselves on food-like substances, and we cannot (and should not) continue to neglect our bodies and our health. And if you don't see why, and are solidly stuck in your own eating habits, here's the deal clincher: optimum nutrition can help resolve your tinnitus and prevent it from reoccurring in the future. What else do you need to know?

Instead of filling up on garbage, we need to make healthy food choices and nourish our bodies with the best, high-quality food that is out there.

Great nutrition supports your body and your mind. It boosts your immune system, helps your body heal illness or injuries, and promotes excellent mental health.

Most importantly for us, it will help you to cope with the symptoms of tinnitus, promote a more positive peaceful mind-set and help your body to heal and your nervous system to return to a more normal restful state.

Background Noise

This is the simplest trick to use in reducing your tinnitus symptoms. Tinnitus often rears its ugly head and becomes more noticeable when your surroundings are quiet, such as at bedtime, in the bathroom, in the public library, when studying, or when focusing on certain tasks.

Use background sounds such as music, the radio, the TV or even "white" noise to conceal the tinnitus, reduce stress, and distract you from your symptoms. If you suffer from a milder form, you may find this eliminates your symptoms all together.

Weight Loss: Overcoming Overweight and Obesity

It's often in vogue for vegans to proclaim to others that their vegan diet is the optimal key to amazing success when it comes to weight loss. It's also true that people have many great reasons to believe that the vegan lifestyle will melt off those pounds. Generally, we vegans really *are* slimmer than most meat-eaters, and we also usually consume a much lower quantity of fat and sugar in our diets than do meat-eaters. In fact, much research has shown that following a plant-based diet is a lifestyle that is linked to a lower body weight.

Statistics also have shown that people who eat a meat-laden diet generally have the highest body weight for their age, whereas in comparison, vegans in the same age groups usually have much lower body weights. In fact, on average, vegans are roughly thirty pounds lighter than their meat-eating counterparts. Thirty pounds is a significant amount of weight! It can mean the difference between looking down and seeing your toes—or not. (A protruding stomach can take that choice away.) Adopting a vegan lifestyle can also lead to a significant drop in your body mass index (BMI), which is the height and weight measurement that is used by most doctors to determine whether people are of normal size, overweight, obese, or, at the worst, morbidly obese, which is really, really fat.

However, at the same time, it is very important to realize that the idea that you can merely eliminate meat from your diet and you will then inevitably transform into a supermodel-esque size zero—well, this is a myth. It's just not going to happen. There's a lot more that goes into adjusting the overall BMI equation downward than by simply ending your meat reliance, namely, weight loss also means you need to take a hard look at your nonmeat food choices too. For example, it's still possible (and is common in some teenagers) to be a *chubby* vegan simply because of very poor food choices. As we saw earlier in this chapter when we talked about health, you need to be mindful about what you eat and to avoid turning to nonmeat junk food options.

It's also important to know that some experts believe that food preservatives and other food additives may be "obesogenic"—an invented word that means that such foods may be obesity inducing. This means that these experts believe that when some ingredients are added to food, these additives may significantly trigger a greater risk for obesity than would be present without consuming those same additives. For example, some research indicates that sodium benzoate, a preservative that is found in many packaged salad dressings, may decrease the production of leptin. Leptin is a natural substance that your body makes to control your fat storage and less leptin is a bad thing.

Other food additives may be obesogenic. Researchers such as Amber L. Simmons and colleagues' reported in a 2014 issue of *Current Obesity Reports* that the chemical mono-oleoylglycerol (MOG) may affect a person's lipid levels. MOG is a substance that is used as an emulsifier in ice cream, whipped cream, shortening, peanut butter, chocolate, frozen desserts, and many other products. An emulsifier prevents ingredients such as oil from separating out from the other ingredients.

Have you ever noticed that you have to stir up natural peanut butter to get it back into the thick and sticky condition loved by so many? You don't have to stir up emulsified peanut butter since it constantly remains in the same thickened condition because of food additives. But if experts are right about additives triggering obesity, then that spoonful of supermarket peanut butter may cost you more than many calories it contains. Instead, you could be unknowingly escalating your appetite. Yikes!

Much more research needs to be done on food additives and preservatives and their risk for triggering obesity in consumers, as well as their risks for causing other possible health problems. But here's the bottom line: it makes sense that if you drop sketchy foods from your diet, particularly the prepackaged foods and junk foods you can buy at the nearest convenience store, then at least some of your weight loss may stem from avoiding the chemicals found in these obesogenic foods.

Another tip: Be forewarned about "diet" foods. (And be sure to also warn your teenager if you have one). These supposedly low-calorie items that are available in supermarkets, pharmacies, and at many other sites, may be full of fat and high in calories, depending on how much you eat. This is especially a problem when consumers ignore the recommended portion size on the food label, as most people do. For example, a quick glance at a bag of diet candy or diet cookies may seem to indicate there are only a few calories in the product. However, if you actually take the time to read the package label, you might discover—to your major dismay—that those scant number of calories listed on the label actually refer to eating just one or two candies or maybe three cookies.

Eat the whole bag, and a person may as well splurge on a large shake at McDonald's! (Don't do that either!) The best advice is, whenever possible, *avoid* all prepackaged foods, diet or otherwise. And if you do eat them, read the label first to find out what the portion size is, especially for the "low-calorie" portion!

It's best to eat whole, nutrient-dense food and consume organic fruits and vegetables, so that eventually your waistline will reap the many wonderful benefits of the vegan diet!

Better Mood and Energy

No doubt about it, following a vegan lifestyle can result in a better mood, more energy, and greater feelings of calm and happiness. When we feed our bodies with the right kind of healthy and nutritious foods, we don't just feel the physical benefits. Rather, the healthy state of our bodies contributes to our mental and emotional well-being, as well as making us feel better and happier overall. Fueling our bodies with the right kind of food can boost our energy levels as well, since our bodies have to work less hard to rid ourselves of the junk in our systems. Add to that the knowledge that we, as vegans, are doing our part to make this world a better place, and it really isn't surprising that people who make the switch end up happier overall!

Furthermore, many plant foods contain libido-boosting properties, and vegan diets result in lower body weight that increases the release of sex hormones. This means that the vegan diet can improve your sex life as well, and I'm sure that for many of us, that would be a great reason to be happy!

Increased Life Span

With all of the health benefits and improved feelings that veganism can bring, it's no wonder that veganism can be a great way to prolong our lives. This is strongly supported by research, such as a study conducted on ninety-six thousand people in Canada and the United States that found that vegan men live an average of 9.5 years longer, and vegan women live 6.1 years longer than their meat-eating counterparts.

The trend extends to those who haven't completely eliminated meat from their diets too. For example, semivegetarians who only consume meat once a week, as well as pescatarians, have been found to have increased protection against some diseases.

A thirty-year study on the residents of Okinawa, Japan, revealed that the secret to their long lives (residents of the area have among the highest life expectancies in the world) were the staples of their diet, which included fruits, vegetables, complex carbohydrates, and soy.

The conclusion is simple, really: the vegan lifestyle doesn't just improve the quality of life, but it helps people live longer too, and who doesn't want that?

Now that we've had a good run through of the many health benefits that the vegan lifestyle can bring, let's move on to some of the other major reasons why making the switch is the right choice!

Animal Cruelty

There are no two ways about it: eating meat causes animals to suffer. Period. This isn't something people can argue over or brush under the carpet (although the majority of us try to do just that). Animals suffer horrendously, not only through both their treatment when they are alive, but also in the manner of their death. In the United States alone, over eight billion animals are killed for food each and every year. That's a whole lot of suffering. Do you know what actually goes on behind closed doors? You only need to take an hour from your day to watch one of the many documentaries out there that cover the meat industry to find out just how hellish it really is.

In the meantime, imagine if you spent your days packed tightly into a tiny cage or pen, unable to take a single step your entire life, unable to turn around or bend over and touch your toes. You're left vulnerable to epidemic after epidemic, and there's no medical care in sight for you or any of the countless poor souls that share your fate. If you die, others will just end up trampling all over you, and those in charge will simply toss your poor carcass aside without a second thought. There's no nourishing, life-giving sunlight warming your skin, no fresh air filling your lungs, no much-needed medical care, and definitely no exercise.

No, I'm not talking about barbaric war crimes, or any rituals practiced by ancient civilizations. This is how we treat the animals in our factory food chain right here, right now.

Before you tell me that I'm deluded, and that it doesn't matter because animals don't have feelings, think again. Any pet owner will be able to tell you the astonishing depth of feeling and character that animals can show. What makes our pets any different from other animals raised solely for food? Aren't they all animals—living, breathing parts of this earth—just the same?

If you object and tell me that there are countless free-range farms out there, and that there are "kinder" ways of producing meat, think yet again. Free-range doesn't always mean what we think it does. Free range only means that the animals have access to green space, but not that they are free to roam. Free range and farm-raised don't tell us anything. Those poor animals still end up the same way: dead and bleeding. So is it any wonder that more and more of us are turning away from this cruelty and toward the peaceful, kind life of veganism?

Animals are not ours to use as we please, and we can all do our part to end this suffering, first and foremost, by ending our support for the meat industry and changing the way we look at food.

Natural Reasons

Nearly all vegans seek to actively avoid foods that they know are jam-packed with artificial additives and preservatives because they realize that these products could be harmful to their health and to the health of their children. As mentioned earlier, some research studies also indicate that these items may make you fat. Preservatives and food additives are often found in so-called ready-made foods, and these products are frequently microwaved or otherwise prepared within minutes. To ensure that such foods are available on demand at any given time, convenience food items are usually full of preservatives that stave off the spoiling that would otherwise occur. Food preservatives are chemicals that are added to foods to prevent the food from spoiling over time by exposure to the air, molds, fungi, and other intrusions that could cause food contamination.

Three common food preservatives are butylated hydroxyanisole (BHA), butylated hydroxytoluene (BHT), and ethylenediaminetetraacetic acid (EDTA). These preservatives with long names are used often in preserving processed foods. Other food preservatives include calcium sorbate, sodium nitrate, sodium benzoate, potassium sorbate, sodium erythorbate, ascorbic acid, and calcium propionate.

It's also true that additives that are not preservatives are often included in foods for a variety of reasons. For example, some additives artificially enhance the flavor of some foods, while others provide a particular desired color. Cola soft drinks (either diet or sugar-filled) would not be brown without added coloring, and margarine wouldn't be yellow without yellow dye. Some additives artificially thicken products or keep them crispy for a longer period than would occur without their use.

As with most major issues in the country, there is a government agency in charge of food preservatives and food additives. It's the Food and Drug Administration (FDA), a federal agency. The FDA also maintains a database of more than three thousand food ingredients entitled "Everything Added to Food in the United States (EAFUS)" which can be found at the following site:

https://www.fda.gov/food/food-additives-petitions/substances-added-food-formerly-eafus

Some of the food items listed by the FDA are simple and generally accepted by many people, like flour or baking soda, while others are chemicals with complicated names.

It may (or may not) surprise you that the FDA reports that some food additives are entirely exempt from government regulation. There are two primary types of food additives that fit this category, according to the FDA, including additives in either group I or group II. The additives in group I were used prior to 1958, and the government considers them safe to use now in the twenty-first century. Group I entries include such items as the chemicals potassium nitrate and sodium nitrate that are used to preserve processed lunch meats. (Many health experts may differ about the relative healthiness of these additives.) Moving on to group II, the additives in this list are generally recognized as safe by the FDA, either because of their use before 1958 or based on safety that was demonstrated in past research studies. Monosodium glutamate (MSG) is a flavor additive that is found in group II.

More on Food Preservatives

Preservatives are used in numerous food products. Here are a few examples of such products: packaged cereals, packaged salad dressings, snack foods, fruit jellies, and many different beverages. If you want to avoid food preservatives, then you need to avoid all processed foods. In fact, you and your family will be much better off, health-wise, if you *do* follow this practice. Processed foods also include the snack foods that too many people buy at supermarkets, like chips and dips.

Other Food Additives

As mentioned earlier, some additives change the color of a broad array of different food products, including jams and jellies, canned pie fillings, and many kinds of cheese. There are nine different colors that are certified by the FDA. One color, FD&C Yellow 5, has been found to cause hives in a few people (an estimated one in ten thousand people).

Hives is an allergic skin reaction that causes a sudden and often very itchy breakout, which can feel like you're covered with fleas. Some children are sensitive to tartrazine, the synthetic yellow dye that is found in FD&C Yellow 5. The law requires that when this food additive is present, it must be included on the product label. In this manner, people who are hypersensitive to this yellow dye may avoid products that include it.

Some added colors are exempt from certification by the FDA because they are derived from vegetables or other natural substances. For example, grape skin extract is an exempt food additive (used to create the colors red and green), as is dehydrated beet, which creates bluish-red to brown colors in food products.

Food additives are also employed to improve the appearance of some foods or to control their acidity. Acidity levels are controlled in frozen desserts, chocolate, and some canned foods. The types of products used to control acidity are sodium carbonate, lactic acid, and ammonium hydroxide. There are also food additives that are used in bread and other baked goods in order to stimulate the action of yeast.

Ammonium phosphate and calcium sulfate are two key chemicals used for this purpose.

Food additives aren't all inherently bad, but it's important to be aware of what additives are included in the foods that you and your family eat.

Environmental Reasons

Modern farming methods are irreparably damaging the environment and destroying the world which we live in, and intensive meat production is primarily responsible for this. Our ancestors farmed in a way that was sustainable, in tune with nature, and respectful of the planet. Today, however, we rape the land for what it can provide without heeding the consequences. We take and take from the earth, without ever giving back or thinking of the damage we cause, so much so that our children's children may end up living in a world completely unrecognizable from what it is today. Here are just some of the effects that the endless greed from the meat industry causes:

Pollution Harms the Environment and Hurts Animals and People: Considering Pesticides

Herbicides, fungicides, and pesticides are frequently sprayed on crops, many of which are ultimately destined to become animal feed. Other pesticides are sprayed to destroy the insects that would devour the crops and impede the subsequent arrival of fruits and vegetables to local supermarkets nationwide.

Pesticides are more commonly used than herbicides, and the Centers for Disease Control and Prevention (CDC) says that in considering all pesticides, more than a billion pounds of pesticides are used every year in the United States. In addition, there are more than seventeen thousand different products that are used as pesticides by Americans. Pesticides are used to kill cockroaches, ants, spiders, and other insects that are found in homes or businesses nationwide. They are also used to kill rats, fleas, and ticks.

Although pesticides are often used to destroy insects, the reality is that their effects and influence often extend much further beyond the local area and into other habitats far from the local area where these pesticides were sprayed or otherwise dispersed. Pesticides can harm the ecosystem of animals in these surrounding environments, as well as ride roughshod over the plant life of the area. Even the fish in the ocean are affected by pesticides.

Pesticides also are known to change microscopic protons that are known as prions. This effect interferes with the DNA of all forms of life, and consequently, the use of pesticides may lead to the development of diseases like mad cow disease.

How Pesticides Are Harmful

Pesticide use destroys the topsoil of the environment, and then it seeps through the ground and into the local water supply, causing contamination of fresh water. These toxic materials further poison the local wildlife, kill the fish, and damage or destroy many delicately balanced ecosystems.

Consider the Honeybee

Not all insects are or should be automatically considered undesirable. For example, many researchers are currently concerned about the harmful effects of pesticides on the honeybee population in the United States and other countries. Pesticides kill some of these bees or, if the bees live, the chemicals act to harm their immune systems, making the bees weaker and significantly more susceptible to disease.

Honeybees are surprisingly important in the food chain for both animals and people. In addition to producing their delicious honey, honeybees also aid in the pollination of many foods that are needed by all living creatures. Their key contribution lies in their pollination activities. These bees transfer pollen from one part of a plant to another part, thus enabling the growth of fruits, nuts, vegetables, and flowers. Some examples of the foods that are pollinated with the aid and assistance of the honeybee are cantaloupes, cherries, blueberries, almonds, apples, and pumpkins, and there are many more.

High and Low-Risk Pesticide-Exposed Fruits and Vegetables

Experts from the United States Department of Agriculture (USDA) and the FDA together have researched the percentage of pesticides on many fruits and vegetables, and have reported that some fruits and vegetables in the United States are particularly at risk for having a high exposure to the residual pesticide. For example, the researchers found that nearly all (99 percent) of apples included pesticides. Other examples of produce that tested high in pesticides included strawberries, raspberries, celery, potatoes, and tomatoes.

In contrast, some fruits and vegetables have a significantly *low* exposure to residual pesticides, including avocadoes, sweet potatoes, pineapples, onions, eggplant, and grapefruit. Therefore, if you need to purchase fruits or vegetables in a supermarket rather than buying organic, then go with the lower-risk items. Choose the sweet potatoes over the potatoes or the pineapple over the apple.

Meat and Pesticides

Experts report that meat contains fourteen times more pesticides than plant food! That's incredible, but the situation gets much worse—farms also give their animals that are grown for food other products, such as growth hormones, antibiotics, salts, and heavy metals. (Yet another reason to avoid eating meat.) All of these items together further pollute the surrounding lands. If a new vegan has difficulty giving up meat, there are many other options such as soy or tofu, and there are many great vegan recipes that will please the choosiest palate!

Pesticides Are Harmful to Humans

In addition to hurting the environment, pesticides can also be harmful to humans, and the CDC says that the average person carries remnants of nearly thirty different pesticides within the body. The World Health Organization (WHO) has also stated that nearly a quarter million people worldwide die from pesticide poisoning every year. Many of these deaths occur in developing countries that have few or no safety regulations. However, pesticides also harm people living in developed countries. For example, farmworkers in the United States are particularly at risk for harm from pesticide use.

The CDC says there are about two million farmworkers in the United States, and each year, farmworkers suffer from up to twenty thousand pesticide poisonings that are diagnosed by doctors. These are the cases that doctors actually identify—it's likely there are less severe cases that are *not* identified by doctors.

Some symptoms of a dangerous exposure to pesticides may include the following:

- Memory loss
- Visual problems
- Unstable mood
- Poor coordination
- Nausea and vomiting
- Photosensitivity (light sensitivity)
- Confusion

Pesticide exposure can lead to infertility, cancer, and hormonal problems, and also may cause harm to a developing fetus. People who have been exposed to pesticides and who show any symptoms should be sure to consult with their physician.

Children and Pesticide Effects

Sadly, children are the most vulnerable people to be harmed by pesticides, and even a small amount of pesticide exposure can lead to sickness and chronic long-term problems in children. Studies of children born to mothers who were exposed to organophosphates (a popular category of insecticide) have shown that the mothers' high exposure to these substances was significantly linked to lower intelligence quotients in their children. In addition, prenatal exposure to organophosphates has been found to be associated with a decrease in a child's perceptual reasoning.

Research also has demonstrated that children between the ages of eight to fifteen years who showed high urinary levels of exposure to organophosphates also suffered double the risk for developing attention deficit hyperactivity disorder (ADHD) when they were compared with children with low or no exposure to organophosphates.

In 2012, the American Academy of Pediatrics (AAP) published a policy statement on pesticide exposure in children. This prestigious organization noted that many children are exposed to pesticides every day, and that children also have "unique susceptibilities to their potential toxicity." Of course, acute poisoning is the most serious risk for children, but chronic exposure to pesticides is also dangerous. The AAP recommended that pediatricians ask parents about pesticide use in or near their homes, and the organization also advised doctors to recommend the least toxic methods of pesticide use.

Some research indicates that pesticide exposure may lead to obesity in children, although the mechanism for how this may happen is unknown.

Biological Pesticides

Some pesticides are called "biological" pesticides, or biopesticides, and these types of pesticides are generally considered much safer than traditional pesticides. Biological pesticides are used by organic farmers, but they are also increasingly used by traditional growers. What are they? Biopesticides are naturally-derived substances that repel insects, such as citronella, garlic, and many other substances. Although bugs may hate them, these substances are not harmful to animals or humans, nor are they risky for the environment. The Environmental Protection Agency (EPA) reported in 2015 that their agency has registered more than 430 active biological agents, and they have also awarded grants for further research on the production of biopesticides. The EPA estimates that more than eighteen million acres of farmland were treated with biopesticides in 2012—and that figure is probably significantly higher now.

Going Organic

For now, it's still probably best to avoid traditional supermarket produce whenever possible because these products are likely to contain organophosphates that may linger on, and washing doesn't always rinse away all the insecticide. (And, often, children and some adults are not very thorough about washing their fruit or vegetables in the first place!) The best practice is to buy organic produce because, as mentioned earlier, these growers will not use harmful pesticides. Experts estimate that by going organic, you can reduce your pesticide exposure by as much as eighty percent. You may not be able to avoid all pesticides, but an eighty percent decrease is an excellent change for the better.

Deforestation

Our forests (especially rainforests) are precious, yet we are clearing land for meat production at an astonishing rate, which seems to show no signs of slowing. The areas of cleared land are used for cattle ranching (grazing) or growing cattle feed, and you'd be surprised to find out how extensive the deforestation has been in the name of the cattle industry. In fact, according to Greenpeace, ten million hectares of rainforest have been cleared in the Brazilian Amazon for cattle ranching between 1996 and 2006. Take note, in a mere decade, they've cleared an area that's roughly the size of Portugal! And that's just in Brazil. Imagine how many hectares of forest lands have been cleared around the world in the decades since cattle ranching first became a major industry. Do you still think the meat people put on their plates is worth all of those costs? Probably not.

Erosion and the Degradation of Soil Health

What you take from the land, you must give back: that's the ancient wisdom that has enabled us to sustain thousands of generations on our lands and continues to do so. Yet, modern industrial farms think they are above this wisdom. Their arrogance and disregard for nature are harming the soil itself. Honest farmers know that you must rest the land you are farming and rotate crops to replenish the soil and let it fertilize in a natural way. Intensive farmers don't do this; they simply don't care. They keep too many animals, don't give back to the land, and wonder why the soil is losing nutrients and water.

CO_2 Production

The beef industry produces huge amounts of carbon dioxide (CO_2), more so in fact than beef-free, vegan, or vegan diets. It's a proven fact that 18 percent of global carbon emissions come from the beef industry, and as we all know, increasing CO_2 levels are harmful to the environment. It might interest you to know that a vegan's carbon footprint is around half that of a meat-eater's.

If we want to take concrete action against these large and greedy industries that threaten nature, then one of the best ways of doing so is starting with ourselves and how we live our lives. By adopting a vegan lifestyle, we cut our support for these industries and do our part in ensuring that future generations get to enjoy the same beautiful earth that we've experienced.

Religious and Spiritual Reasons

Many organized and personal religions around the world believe that it is intrinsically wrong to eat meat and actively promote a cruelty-free vegan diet. These include Jainism, Hinduism, and Buddhism.

Jainism demands that its followers adopt a diet and lifestyle that is 100 percent free from suffering, whereas Hinduism and Buddhism leave the choice to the follower, though they do encourage people to choose kinder and healthier ways of eating.

It's not just religions that aim to avoid lifestyles that promote suffering and death. Leading figures from many world religions have stood up and have sung the praises of a vegan diet. The truth of the matter is that many religions advocate caring for our own bodies, compassion for those around us, and being responsible for the welfare of the gift of nature that we have been given. Veganism addresses each of these quite soundly, so it's no surprise that veganism shares many ties with spiritual ways of living too!

Economic Reasons

It also costs less to eat a vegan diet than a meat diet. Face it, meat is expensive. In fact, meat accounts for a hefty portion of American food budgets. When I walk along the aisles of my local supermarket, it always amazes me to see just how much meat costs. Vegetables, on the other hand, are much, much cheaper, and for the health benefits that come with eating veggies, you simply can't get a better deal elsewhere! Think about it. Poorer and developing nations around the world thrive on simple diets based around rice and beans. Why can't we? Plus, if we ate a veggie diet, then we'd have a few extra dollars at the end of the week to treat ourselves to something awesome! Replacing the nearly two hundred pounds of meat that the average nonvegan person consumes every year with healthier and more budget-friendly plant-based foods can lower your food expenses by about $4,000 a year, and that doesn't even include all of the money you're saving on the medical bills you're avoiding, thanks to your healthier lifestyle. I don't know about you, but all of that extra money in my pocket sounds pretty awesome to me!

As you can see, we are driven to become vegans for many differing reasons, and these reasons can grow and merge as time goes on. One of my closest friends turned to veganism for health reasons in the beginning, but discovering more about the welfare and environmental issues behind veganism made him stick with this way of eating. Nowadays, he educates others using his newfound knowledge. You can do so too, and it all starts with beginning your journey into veganism, which I'll discuss in the next chapter.

Chapter 4

Getting Started on a Vegan Diet

MOST PEOPLE THINK that getting into veganism is as easy as ditching the meat and munching on green leafy foods. In reality, though, it's not as simple as that. As amazing as the benefits of going vegan may be, many will run into challenges and difficulties in making such a major adjustment in their lives for the first time. Thankfully, there is a goldmine of information available from those who have been in your situation before, and that can make the shift a lot easier for you. Here are some tips that I've gathered from my own experiences to make the start of your vegan journey that much smoother and easier to stick to.

Be Kind to Yourself and Find What Works For You

Perhaps the most important thing to remember about starting your new vegan lifestyle is that the journey is never the same for any two people. Different things work for different people, and your goal is to find what works for you, since that's exactly what could make the difference between sticking to your decision to go vegan, or just giving up and going back to your old ways.

Still, if you do end up slipping, or "falling off the horse," so to speak, that's perfectly fine. You're only human, after all, and, as I've said, every journey is different. Of course, that includes slipups too!

Some people will pick up the vegan diet like a duck takes to water, while others will struggle more, and that's just the way it is.

So be kind to yourself and always remember that what's important is that you pick yourself up, dust yourself off, and get right back into it every single time you fall. If you find you're having difficulty with that, it helps to remember what drove you to make the switch in the first place, and the awesome rewards that await you once you've truly made the vegan lifestyle your own.

Start Slow

For people who have been eating meat their whole lives, going vegan may appear to be quite a daunting task. Drastically changing something as important as your daily diet can be quite a struggle, but who says you have to make the change overnight? If going completely vegan is turning out to be more difficult than you first expected, try starting off slowly, taking a step-by-step approach to your transition.

You could try having a veggie-only day once a week, and then, once you've gotten more used to it, gradually increase that to twice a week, then thrice a week, and so on, until your daily diet has become completely vegan.

Alternatively, you could also start by dropping one type of meat first, like pork or beef, before going on to drop chicken, fish, and all the other meats, one at a time.

If things are turning out to be especially challenging, you could even try vegan meat substitutes to ease your transition even more. Although they aren't the most ideal thing to get used to, several shops now offer plant-based meat substitutes meant to feel and taste like the real thing, without the associated guilt. Some of these substitutes, however, undergo greater amounts of processing than more natural foods, which is something you would probably want to avoid in the long run. So it's probably best if these were used as a stepping stone toward truly healthy eating, rather than as a long-term solution.

The crucial thing to remember is that if you start off slow, it isn't a shame at all, nor does it make you any less of a vegan. What's important is that you find the way that works best for yourself so that you can begin consistently reaping the benefits of a vegan diet for the rest of your life!

Make It Enjoyable (By Testing New Recipes and Trying New Things)

Another thing that can make the shift to veganism challenging is that, for some, it might not be very fun at first. For people who are used to some of the intense flavors and distinct textures that come with the experience of eating meat, a sudden shift to veganism can leave them missing what they used to have every day. Add to that the fact that you won't instantly feel the improvements of your new healthy lifestyle after just one or two days, as well as the possibility that your own thoughts and feelings might be influenced by the common misconception of vegan food being bland, and you could end up perceiving sticking to your new vegan diet as a chore, rather than the life-changing improvement that it really is. Thankfully, there are a number of ways around this problem that will have you happily living your new healthy lifestyle in no time!

As mentioned earlier in the book, in the chapter on the common myths and misconceptions about veganism, vegan life is brimming with a variety of healthy options, and the sky is the limit in terms of the possibilities. Besides periodically having some of those meat substitutes, the answer could just lie in how you approach the challenge. Treat it like a game that encourages improvisation and where the objective is to try out as many new things as possible to find what you really like. Pull those cookbooks off your shelves and dive right in! (You could also purchase one of the many vegan cookbooks available now.) There are many delicious flavors that you probably haven't tried or even thought of yet, so experiment! Make your start in the journey to veganism as enjoyable as it can be by trying something new every day. Experiment with different dishes, tweak some recipes, and surprise yourself! You never know you might just find that perfect taste you've been looking for all this time, and you'll even be able to call it your own!

If you're looking for a place to start, here's a top tip: try playing around with beans and lentils. As a vegan, they'll be your new best friend: they're a rich source of many vitamins and minerals, they taste great, and they can add bite to any dish while being very versatile!

Make It Social!

Any major change in life can be frightening, but being around people who understand what you're going through and who can empathize with you always makes things better. Having the right company is never a bad thing, so why not try making the switch together with some close friends or family members? You can challenge each other, share tips and recipes, and celebrate milestones together!

If you're having trouble finding people to share your journey with, try going online! There are dozens upon dozens of online forums and blogs out there dedicated to the vegan lifestyle, where people regularly share their thoughts, experiences, tips, and just about anything veganism-related with each other. If you enjoy writing, try starting your own blog as well. You'll be able to write about your daily experiences, and you can look back later on and see how you've progressed. You can also even share your thoughts and feelings with other interested and like-minded people.

As that old Beatles song goes, "I get by with a little help from my friends," and starting a vegan lifestyle is no different.

Connecting with other people and sharing your journey with friends can make it all more worthwhile and fulfilling in the end, so get on out there and be social!

Plan Ahead

Another source of issues for many beginner vegans is the unforeseen practical problems one might encounter from day-to-day. There's no doubt about it, adhering to a vegan lifestyle does require some degree of planning.

For most people, this means making sure that you have enough vegan food available to you wherever you may be, and that you minimize any temptations you might run into along the way. After all, you definitely do not want to be caught miles out from home with only steaks or burgers as your last remaining food options, or maybe find that you've ditched the poultry completely only to see mouth-watering leftover thanksgiving turkey calling to you from the back of a family member's fridge, begging to be eaten.

Plan carefully, try to guess any potential stumbling blocks, and get yourself organized accordingly. It's like giving up smoking in many ways—you need to have an action plan if you want it to work. List places where you can get a quick vegan fix in your area (or wherever you might be heading to if you plan to spend any time away from home, for that matter). Always be prepared, and it's almost guaranteed that your switch to veganism will go much, much smoother.

Know What to Do When Eating Out

Related to planning ahead is being prepared for all the possibilities that might come along whenever you eat out. While home-cooked dishes for me will always win out over restaurant food, you might want a change of scenery from time to time, and there's also no telling when your friends are going to come knocking at your door, trying to drag you out for a night in town. Although there are some vegan restaurants out there that cater to our plant-based needs, there's no telling when life's demands might bring you to nonvegan restaurants, so here are a few tips on eating out vegan-style.

As mentioned earlier, planning ahead is key, and a large part of that is picking a vegan restaurant to eat at, or making sure that there are restaurants in whatever area you might be heading to that can cater to your needs. Thankfully, there are many online resources that provide great lists of vegan-friendly restaurants in your area, or anywhere around the world, when you're traveling. So it's really just as easy is logging on, finding a destination, and heading over! What's more, many of these online resources also include restaurant reviews, making it even easier for you to decide where (and where not) to eat!

If you ever do find yourself in a nonvegan restaurant, though, there are some things that you need to look out for, as it's never really as simple as finding the meatless dishes on the menu, ordering them, and then chowing down. If you've been on a vegan diet for quite some time, your stomach may not agree with some of the dishes that look completely safe at face value. If you're ordering fried dishes, for instance, make sure to always ask the waiter about the oil they use for cooking, and whether or not the dish you're ordering shares the same oil used in cooking chicken, pork, steak, or other meats.

Several years ago, I had an experience while visiting Las Vegas, Nevada. It was a hot, sunny morning, and out of convenience, I decided to stop by Nathan's, the east coast chain restaurant, for some breakfast. As usual, the choices for vegans were limited, so I just decided to have what appeared to be the safest items on the menu: toast and hash browns. As I sat eating my food, however, all of a sudden, I began to feel the strong urge to throw up. I felt sick, and it's almost like my body didn't want anything to do with the food I was having.

Of course, at first, I couldn't for the life of me figure out why it was happening then, but when I ended up at Nathan's again, sometime later, it all made sense. It was the oil. I noticed the cook putting bacon in the same fryer he used to make my hash browns, and I realized that after so many years without meat, my body reacted to those hash browns as if they were something foreign in my body.

Even dishes that actually sell themselves as "vegan" or that use the term "vegetable" aren't always safe, either. Another time, I was at a Panda Express where I stop by a lot to order the vegetable fried rice and vegetable spring rolls. Now these were dishes that I'd already enjoyed many times before, and they even had the word "vegetable" in their names, so what could go wrong, right? Well, that one time, after eating my meal, my stomach inexplicably began to hurt. As it turns out, similar to my experience at Nathan's, the oil used for cooking the vegetable spring rolls and the vegetable fried rice was the same oil they used for cooking their meats.

With nonvegan restaurants, you can never really be too sure, so don't ever think twice about asking the waiter! While it may be embarrassing at first to have to feel like the annoying customer who asks too many questions, that's probably the last thing you'll be thinking about when it's all too late, and you're already doubled over in pain and sick to your stomach. In the end, what's truly important is that you get the food that you need, nothing more, nothing less.

If there are vegetables available on the menu, make sure to ask the waiter whether those dishes have any animal by- products of any sort in them. Some dishes, although technically meatless, do contain these by-products, and they may end up giving you an upset stomach or making you feel guilty about what you had just eaten.

It took me years, for example, to find out that gelatin is processed by using bones and connective tissues from animals. I was in shock when I found out that my favorite dessert, gelatin topped off with whipped cream, was made with animals. Although I was fortunate enough not to ever have experienced an upset stomach after eating gelatin, I do take my vegan lifestyle seriously and have stayed away from gelatin since. It's all about sticking to your principles, and my principles definitely won out over my love for gelatin.

For another tip, I find that a great way of enjoying a meal out with friends is to eat before you head out and then simply order a lighter vegetable dish, such as baked potato, once you get to the restaurant. That way, you can at least be sure that you won't end up hungry out of a lack of options, and if your stomach somehow doesn't agree with what you had just eaten, then at least it won't be in as bad of a position as if you had consumed a heavy full meal. If you want to be absolutely sure about what you'll be having, though, home-cooked meals are simply the best way to go, and packing food for yourself is always an option.

Make Sure You Get All the Nutrients You Need

As wonderful as the health benefits of a vegan diet are, another very important thing to pay attention to is getting all of the nutrients you need. While many people presume that veganism is the highway to good health, they are only getting part of the bigger picture.

The unfortunate truth is that strictly adhering to a specific diet can leave people with a deficiency in certain nutrients. Since veganism can involve very strict and demanding diets, many people who enter into veganism without properly educating themselves run the risk of developing nutrient deficiencies.

In the next chapter, I'll be discussing how things can go wrong, and how you can avoid problems by identifying those nutrients that may cause a deficiency in typical vegan diets, as well as how you might be able to properly fulfill these nutrient-related needs.

Chapter 5

Where It All Went Wrong For Me and How You Can Avoid It (My Story Of Nutrient Deficiency)

To be perfectly honest, I was one of those people who made the mistake of not keeping track of the nutrients that my body needs. I am a vegan, and it very nearly killed me. To make matters worse, it was entirely my fault and could have easily been avoided. Here is my story.

My life was pretty awesome just before it happened: I was (relatively) young, full of energy, and living life to the fullest. I had been a vegan for about twelve years, and I loved every second of it!

All of a sudden, though, things began to change. The most noticeable difference was my energy level: it really took a nosedive. Now, I love keeping myself busy; so being the kind of person I was, I just put it down to working too hard and spending too many nights burning the candle at both ends and assumed it would resolve itself in time after I'd had the opportunity to rest.

Then the headaches came. These debilitating headaches would restrict me to my bed for days on end, and they also came with chills that would keep me buried under mountains of blankets even in the depths of summer. My symptoms were accompanied by terrible nausea that would leave me helpless and vomiting. "Ahh, so this is what the flu feels like," I said to myself, and so I took it easy once again, thinking that things would get better in a week or two. Boy, was I wrong.

Two months later, I still wasn't getting any better. In fact, things were getting much, much worse, and I was starting to become really concerned. I then crawled off to my doctor in search of hope and a few answers, thinking that he'd give me a prescription for some meds and send me home with orders to take better care of myself. Of course, as these stories usually go, it definitely didn't turn out to be as simple as that. I'll never forget the moment when he broke the life-changing news to me.

I wasn't suffering from the flu. I wasn't even suffering from some kind of strange virus. It was much worse than that. I was suffering from pernicious anemia or an inability to create enough red blood cells due to a lack of vitamin B12, and the prognosis was definitely bleak.

You see, while I thought I was eating a supremely healthy vegan diet, I had actually been depriving my body of vitamin B12, and as a result, my immune system began to attack its own tissues, causing permanent damage; I'd have to inject B12 for the rest of my life. Without it, I would die.

I was utterly devastated. Nevertheless, I never regretted becoming a vegan. Far from it. I had become vegan for all of the right reasons, and I still stood—and, to this day, stand—by them all. However, what I did regret was my ignorance about the damage that a vitamin deficiency could do to my body, and how easily it could have been avoided.

I was naïve, uninformed, and acting solely from the heart, and if I had had someone to guide me, my prognosis could have been a whole lot different, which is one of the main reasons I decided to write this book—to prevent it from happening to you.

Nutrients You Need and Where to Get Them

As you already know, there are several nutrients that might be slightly more challenging to get on a vegan diet, and we need to pay closer attention to them and plan our diets to ensure we are getting them in the right quantities. This chapter will give you a rundown of the core nutrients that you should watch, provide some information on what those nutrients do for your health, and point you toward some great vegetarian and vegan sources for them.

Protein

Protein is one of the necessary ingredients in creating body tissue. It is needed for tissue growth and maintenance and can be found in our skin, muscles, bones, hair, and just about any tissue in the human body you can think of. Protein sometimes also act as a fuel source for the body, for times when carbohydrates (the body's primary source of energy) are not available.

As you can see, proteins are very important in the way our bodies function and are probably one of the most vital nutrients for our bodies. Today, it is recommended that adult males get about 56 grams of protein a day, while adult females should have about 46 grams daily. It is important to note, however, that not all proteins that we consume are exactly the same. You see, proteins are formed by combinations of different amino acids. To avoid a protein deficiency or malnutrition, humans must get enough of each of the different amino acids that our bodies need.

The trouble is while some amino acids can be produced within our bodies, others called essential amino acids can only be found in food sources. Meat and dairy are widely recognized as the best sources of protein, which is why, as vegans, it is important to keep track of our protein intake and to strive to get complete proteins—or proteins that contain enough of each of the amino acids we need—in our diets.

For lacto-ovo vegetarians, here are some great common sources of protein:

- Milk
- Yogurt (especially Greek yogurt, which contains much more protein than regular yogurt)
- Eggs
- Cheese

For vegans, meanwhile, here are the best ways to get your protein:

Complete protein sources

- Chia
- Soy
- Soybeans
- Quorn
- Sprouted grain bread
- Seitan
- Quinoa
- Buckwheat
- Hempseed

Other protein sources:

Seeds

- Chia seeds
- Sunflower seeds
- Poppy seeds
- Sesame seeds
- Pumpkin and squash seeds
- Hemp seeds Flax seeds

Vegetables

- Soybean sprouts
- Lentil sprouts
- Soybeans
- Green peas
- Corn
- Sun-dried tomatoes
- Spinach
- Kale

- Bok choy
- Broccoli
- Cowpeas
- Lima beans
- Brussels sprouts
- Mushrooms
- Artichoke
- Potato
- Asparagus

Soy protein

- Edamame
- Soy milk
- Tofu
- Tempeh
- Soy yogurt

Fruits

- Dried apricots
- Peaches
- Avocado
- Guava
- Prunes
- Dried zante currants
- Dried figs
- Raisins
- Dates
- Passion fruit

Cereal, bread, grains, and pasta

- Quinoa
- Oat bran
- Oats

- Wheat flour
- Whole grain pasta
- Buckwheat Rolled oats
- Couscous
- Bulgur
- Millet (raw)
- Brown rice
- Whole wheat bread and tortillas
- Oatmeal bread
- Rye bread
- Shredded wheat cereal
- Sprouted grain bread

Miscellaneous

- Seitan
- Unsweetened cocoa powder
- Veggie burgers
- Soy protein foods
- Veggie hotdogs
- Hemp

Iron

Iron is the nutrient that produces the hemoglobin which helps red blood cells carry oxygen around our bodies, so you can tell right away how incredibly vital iron is in our everyday lives. The recommended daily intake of iron for men is about 8 mg, while women need about 18 mg a day. If you've noticed the discrepancy between the recommendations for men and women, that's because for women, iron is even more important, especially during times of menstruation and pregnancy, since menstruation depletes the body's iron through blood loss, and also since pregnant women need more iron to meet both their needs and their babies' nutritional needs.

While many associate iron only with meat, it's actually a nutrient that is widely available throughout the plant kingdom. Iron comes in two versions: the meat version (heme iron) and the veggie version (nonheme iron). The difference is that the body absorbs heme iron better than nonheme iron, which means that vegans tend to get less of that important iron. There's no need to be too concerned, though, as there are ways around this problem. We can boost our absorption of iron through consuming vitamin C at the same time by drinking a glass of orange juice with a meal, for instance. It's also good to avoid drinking tea and coffee with your meal, as they reduce the body's absorption of iron. Besides that, paying attention to the food you eat or taking an iron supplement should do the trick.

Still, do keep an eye out for the signs of an iron deficiency, which include lethargy, paleness, fatigue, headaches, chills, and nausea and vomiting. An iron deficiency is no small thing, so if you suspect you might be deficient, please do visit your doctor.

Here are some great vegan sources for iron, grouped according to their type:

Vegetables

- Potatoes
- Sun-dried tomatoes
- Arugula
- Tomato paste
- Cooked spinach
- Peas
- Turnip greens
- Collard greens
- Beet greens
- Swiss chard
- Broccoli

Beans

- Black beans
- Black-eyed peas
- Chickpeas

- Kidney beans
- Lentils
- Lima beans
- Pinto beans
- Tahini
- White beans

Soy

- Tofu
- Spirulina
- Soybeans
- Tempeh

Grains

- Brown rice
- Quinoa
- Oatmeal
- Enriched bagel
- Whole-wheat pasta

Seeds

- Pumpkin seeds
- Fruits
- Dried apricots, Dried peaches
- Prune juice
- Strawberries

Miscellaneous

- Dark chocolate
- Blackstrap molasses
- Dried thyme

Vitamin B12

This vitamin is the source of much controversy within the vegetarian and vegan world. Some say you can get B12 on a vegan diet, while others say you can't. So what is the truth behind all of the discussions?

The answer is not quite straightforward because neither animals nor plants make this vitamin. However, B12 is essential for our health, since humans need 2.4 micrograms daily for cell division and blood formation. Vitamin B12 is produced by bacteria that live in the soil. When animals ingest this soil, the vitamin B12-producing bacteria then inhabit the animals' stomachs and intestines, and those animals, in turn, become sources of the vitamin. While it might not sound very pleasant, it does give us a clue as to why vegans have a harder time getting proper doses of this vitamin.

Since vegans avoid eating the animals that ingest the bacteria-rich soil, we don't get any vitamin B12-rich meat, either, and it is precisely because of these circumstances that I had to suffer through my dietary downfall and now have to inject myself with vitamin B12 for the rest of my life. Had I known about this vitamin's importance, as well as how to get it, then perhaps my prognosis might have been a whole lot different.

Lacto-ovo vegetarians can get their daily dose of vitamin B12 from:

- Fortified soya milk
- Yeast extract
- Brewer's yeast
- Cheese
- Eggs
- Other milk and dairy products

Alternatively, you could also take a high-quality supplement to cover your needs. I can't stress it enough—you really need to ensure you are getting enough B12, since a deficiency could have major repercussions, such as long-term nerve damage, dementia, and pernicious anemia.

Iodine

Iodine is a mineral required so that the thyroid gland can create thyroid hormone, which helps regulate the body's metabolism and aids in the development of the body and its cells, among other things. A deficiency in iodine can lead to hypothyroidism, which can cause fatigue, depression, goiter (thyroid enlargement), weight gain, and intellectual deficiency or impaired brain function.

For vegans, some good sources of iodine are:

- Sea vegetables (such as sea kelp, nori, kombu, wakame, and arame)
- Iodized salt
- Himalayan crystal salt
- Navy beans
- Enriched bread
- Enriched macaroni
- Cream-style corn
- Prunes
- Raisin bran
- Lima beans (boiled)
- Apple juice
- Green peas
- Bananas
- Strawberries
- Green beans
- Cranberries

For lacto-ovo vegetarians, meanwhile, here are some common iodine sources:

- Eggs
- Milk
- Yogurt
- Cheddar cheese

Lastly, here's where pescatarians can get their share of iodine:

- Shrimp
- Canned tuna
- Baked cod
- Lobster

Calcium

Calcium is the "bone nutrient." It's involved in growing new bone and maintaining bone strength, and a deficiency can result in osteoporosis, which leads to brittle bones and fractures. I'm sure that none of that sounds very pretty at all, but the good news is that calcium is a relatively easy mineral to get. With a recommended daily allowance of 1000 mg per day, lacto-ovo vegetarians can get their fill through dairy products, such as milk, yogurt, and cheese, while pescatarians will find salmon to be a great source of calcium.

For vegans, here are some nice sources of calcium:

Soy products

- Soy
- Tempeh
- Tofu
- Edamame

Fruits

- Calcium-fortified orange juice
- Blackberries
- Black currants
- Dried apricots
- Figs
- Dates

Vegetables

- Blackstrap molasses
- Turnip greens (raw)
- Kale (raw)
- Bok choy
- Mustard greens
- Broccoli
- Fennel (raw)
- Arugula
- Artichokes
- Potatoes

Beans

- Tahini
- Garbanzo beans
- Pinto beans
- Black beans
- Great northern beans
- Adzuki beans
- Navy beans

Seeds, nuts, and grains

- Sunflowers seeds
- Almond butter
- Almonds
- Roasted sesame seeds
- Amaranth
- Corn tortillas

Miscellaneous

- Soymilk (fortified with calcium)
- Almond yogurt (fortified with calcium)

- Any fortified non-dairy milk
- Hemp milk

Vitamin D

Vitamin D is calcium's best buddy, and it works closely with calcium to maintain bone health. Vitamin D is very unusual as a vitamin because it acts more like a hormone than a vitamin. As with calcium, vitamin D can be found in dairy products and egg yolks, but these foods are on the bad list of the vegan.

However, our bodies can also produce vitamin D when exposed to the right amount of sunshine. Sadly, this depends on the time of day, the season, and the latitude at which you live, and so many miss out on this magic. If you live in more northern climates, you'd best consider a supplement. The recommended daily allowance is 400 IU for kids and adults up to the age of fifty, and then the allowance increases to 600 for older adults. Be careful, though. An excess of vitamin D can result in an overdose, so please do take good care not to take any more than you need.

Zinc

I'll always remember my father, in his wisdom, popping those round zinc pills at the slightest hint of a cold. The interesting thing was that he always beat the cold much quicker than everyone else around him.

You see, zinc is vital for the immune system, growth, wound healing, hair growth, and even sperm health for men. Luckily, it's one of the easier minerals for vegans to obtain, but only if they're following a decent, whole-food diet. Although there is a wide variety of foods that you can get your zinc from, such as soy, legumes, grains, nuts, and seeds, it is still best to keep an eye on your zinc intake, as phytates, which can be found in some vegan foods, can impede the absorption of the mineral.

In general, some things you can do to improve your zinc intake are to soak your grains before cooking, have a lot of fermented foods, and make sure you get your fill of toasted nuts and seeds too. Also, one quick tip for you: protein improves zinc absorption, so try to combine the two if you can. Below are some great vegan and vegetarian sources of zinc:

Soy foods

- Tofurky Italian sausage (one sausage typically contains 9 mg of zinc)
- Tofu (raw and firm)
- Tempeh
- Edamame

Legumes

- Garbanzo beans
- Pinto beans
- Kidney beans
- Lentils
- Hummus and chickpeas (cooked)

Vegetables

- Mushrooms
- Spinach, broccoli
- Kale
- Corn
- Green peas

Grains

- Wheaties
- Wheat germ cereal
- Rice Chex
- Oatmeal
- Whole-wheat bread

Nuts and seeds

- Almonds
- Cashews
- Chia seeds
- Peanut butter
- Peanuts
- Pecans
- Pistachios
- Pumpkin seeds
- Sunflower seeds
- Walnuts

Miscellaneous

- Miso
- Nutritional yeast

So you see, out of a whole host of vitamins and minerals, we only need to watch our intakes of a handful of them to ensure we are getting what we need. It may sound a bit complicated for now, but it really isn't all that hard. I find the best way is to take a daily vitamin and mineral supplement to cover my bases, while at the same time, topping up with a good wholesome vegan diet. Once you've got all of your nutrients covered, there really isn't much else to fear, so you can focus on taking the next steps in your vegan journey, which I'll discuss in the next section.

Part III

Taking the Next Steps in Veganism

So you've already decided that veganism is the lifestyle for you, and that you want to enjoy all of the healthy benefits that come with such a lifestyle, while doing your part to fight animal cruelty and the destruction of the environment as well. You've taken your first steps into veganism, have learned the basics of the vegan lifestyle, and have educated yourself and covered all your bases when it comes to the nutrients you need. What's next for you? In this part, we discuss the next steps that you can take in your vegan journey to maximize the benefits you receive and to get a more worthwhile and fulfilling experience out of it. You've only scratched the tip of the iceberg, so read on and dive into all of the other benefits that this wonderful lifestyle has to offer!

Chapter 6

Detoxification

WHEN PEOPLE TALK about detoxification and cleansing the body of harmful toxins, it's often seen as a fringe element of veganism. People don't really like to think about harmful toxins building up in their colons or in their arteries, which can often be a by-product of a carnivorous diet. A diet that's high in fat and processed foods tends to slow down our digestive systems, and the elimination or cleansing processes of our bodies are also interrupted.

This can allow harmful bacteria and toxins to accumulate in our systems and can create a general feeling of sluggishness, as well as a host of digestive disorders, such as irritable bowel syndrome or colitis. This is why detoxification is crucial in moving toward a healthier lifestyle. When we begin eating a healthier vegan diet, we start to get more dietary fiber into our systems, and all of a sudden, our digestive systems start to work better.

When you eliminate high-fat meat and processed foods from your diet, then much of your body's energy is freed from the intense work of digesting these foods. Everything becomes clearer—your blood, your organs, and your mind—and you start to become more aware of the toxic nature of the food that you had been eating before.

Toxicity is of much greater concern in the twenty-first century than ever before. There are many new and stronger chemicals abounding, air and water pollution have worsened, and radiation and nuclear power have begun to become another cause for worry. Also, farm animals grown for food are regularly pumped with antibiotics and growth hormones (such as anabolic steroids), which eventually find themselves into human bodies through the consumption of meat, contributing to antibiotic resistance and hormone imbalances in humans. We ingest new chemicals, use more drugs of different kinds, eat more sugar and refined foods, and abuse our bodies daily with various stimulants and sedatives. As a result, the incidence of many toxicity-related conditions has increased over the years. Cancer and cardiovascular disease are two of the main conditions linked with toxicity, and these two alone are already a huge cause for concern.

Besides these two, however, arthritis, allergies, obesity, and many skin problems can also arise, in part due to toxicity. In addition, a wide range of symptoms, such as headaches, fatigue, pains, cough, gastrointestinal problems, and problems from immune weakness, can also all be related to toxicity. When you start a vegan eating plan, your body eventually cleanses itself of the harmful effects of these toxic foods.

While a vegan diet in itself can already do wonders for the human body, there is more to healthy eating and detoxification than just avoiding the meat. To truly detoxify the body, we also need to stay away from junk foods that offer little for our nutrition and from processed food that can often be rife with chemicals, additives, and preservatives. These chemicals, some of which even come from the packaging that our food comes into contact with (such as foils and plastics), find themselves into our meals and can be hazardous to our health and cause a myriad of unforeseen consequences, such as the ingestion of carcinogens and the increased risk of hormonal imbalances. The bottom line is that they're generally unhealthy, so it's best to stay away from them as much as possible. While processed foods and meat substitutes can be useful when taking your first steps toward a true vegan lifestyle thanks to the convenience that they bring, it's still in your body's best interests to move away from them as soon as you can and not make a habit out of consuming them.

If we're supposed to stay away from so many things, then what should we be including in our diets? Well, the answer is really simple: real foods. By real foods, we mean natural foods that come fresh and unprocessed, and, ideally, they are prepared by you. Simply center your diet around these fresh and unprocessed foods and try to cook from scratch whenever you can. Stick to this simple guide, and you'll soon be one step closer to your goal of detoxification and healthy living! A real food diet, after all, delivers to your body exactly what nature intended, with no added garbage. And who can argue with that?

Chapter 7

The Organic Lifestyle

ALTHOUGH AVOIDING PROCESSED foods is definitely the right way to go, some vegans will find that this still isn't enough. Who knows what the produce that we typically find in supermarkets has gone through, after all? Although they may be natural in a sense, and, sometimes, even fresh, there really isn't any way to know where they come from and what's happened to them along the way.

While vegetables are generally great for our bodies, there are still a few things health-conscious eaters might be concerned about, however, and these are genetic modifications and pesticides. Although they are generally marketed as improved versions of our foods, genetically modified organisms, or GMOs, may have negative long-term effects that are still largely unknown at this time. Furthermore, studies have shown a link between GMOs and the increasing number of allergic reactions and digestive disorders experienced by people.

Pesticides provide a much more concrete threat to our well-being. Many of these substances, after all, were designed to kill other living organisms, making it no small wonder that exposure to pesticides has already been linked to a number of medical conditions. The World Health Organization, in fact, states that an estimated three million people per year suffer from some form of pesticide poisoning, which causes about 220,000 deaths annually. Furthermore, perhaps just as concerning are the findings of the Centers for Disease Control and Prevention, or the CDC, that reveal that an estimated twenty-nine different pesticides can be found, on average, in the American body. It sounds terrifying, for sure, doesn't it? But, then again, this is precisely why more and more people have taken things a step further by adopting the organic lifestyle.

But what exactly is the organic lifestyle? In simple terms, the organic lifestyle involves consuming and using natural, organic, and sustainable foods and products, and, essentially, living a life that strives to avoid exposure to harmful chemicals and substances and minimizes the negative impacts of one's actions on the environment.

Products that are "organic" are grown free from any chemical fertilizers or pesticides and are produced without any chemical additives. Farmers who grow organic foods use sustainable practices and steer clear of genetic modifications. You might ask, how do they keep their crops intact, then? Well, to prevent damage from pests and the spread of disease among crops, organic farmers select pest-resistant crops, first and foremost, and also use techniques such as the release of other insects that naturally prey on pests but do not otherwise negatively affect the crops. They also use the strategic planting of smaller crops in key areas with proper spacing. The use of sprays, whether natural or otherwise, comes solely as a last resort, and only when it meets the standards and regulations set by law and by the government agencies tasked with enforcing those standards and regulations—the National Organic Standards Board and the National Organic Program.

Furthermore, to ensure sustainability, organic farmers regularly rotate their crops or switch up the crops that they grow on a given plot of land in different seasons. This allows the nutrients in the soil to naturally replenish, resulting in more fertile land and greater crop yield, and also works to avoid soil erosion and further prevent the accumulation of pests.

This is in stark contrast to conventional farming, which is now widely known to be harmful to the environment. It leads to poor soil and vast areas of deforestation, which then leads to the loss of indigenous birds and animals. In fact, conventional farming methods have had such a severe impact on the environment that some species have become all but eliminated or extinct, thanks to these farming practices.

Without a doubt, this kind of farming has become a massive threat to global biodiversity. There have been huge declines, for instance, in the numbers of bees throughout the world due to the use of pesticides, just as there have been similar declines in bird and animal populations due to deforestation. The deforestation of nature and the destructive farming methods practiced in the meat industry are destroying the habitats of many living species. Since all living things are directly or indirectly connected, little by little, it affects the human population as well.

The ecosystem is a finely tuned network involving numerous organisms, and significant declines in animal populations or the extinctions of entire species can have devastating effects on ecosystems as a whole that can make their effects on humans. As humans, we rely on nature for sustenance, after all, and the extinction of a certain species of fish, for instance, could threaten the food supplies of other animals in the food chain, causing decreases in the populations of these other animals, in turn, possibly leading to food shortages for humans.

For another example of how closely interconnected the different organisms in an ecosystem are, let's look at the bees we mentioned earlier. As we already know, their populations are declining due to the use of pesticides, but what if one day, we all just woke up to find bees extinct? We wouldn't have to worry about bee stings, anymore, that's for sure, but one thing we would have to be very concerned about is our supply of produce. Bees play a big role in one-third of all agricultural food production and are instrumental in the pollination of many plants.

As a result of all of these factors, we know that organic products are safer, healthier, more nutritious, and, in some cases, even better-tasting than their nonorganic counterparts, all the while being environmentally-friendly too. Whatever your reasons may be for adopting a vegan lifestyle—whether health-related or environmentally-minded—organic living has something for you!

It should be noted, however, that not just anyone can try to apply sustainable practices, avoid pesticides, try to grow their crops naturally, and instantly call their products "organic." There are several other product labels out there, and some call their products "natural," which can be quite confusing for people. In reality, all that the label "natural" really means is that genetic modification and synthetic ingredients were avoided, and efforts were made to minimize the processing of the product.

True organic foods on the market that earn the "organic" label have to undergo certification and need to conform to rigid standards set by the Organic Food Protection Act of 1990, as applied and enforced by the government agencies mentioned above—the National Organic Standards Board and the National Organic Program. Even among products that are considered organic, several labels exist to guide consumers. Organic products, for instance, can be "100 percent organic," "organic," "made with organic," or "less than 70 percent organic," with products carrying the "organic" label having 95 percent of its listed ingredients as organic, and products carrying the "made with organic" label containing at least 70 percent organic ingredients.

While it may sound complicated at first, the payoffs of adopting an organic lifestyle are definitely worth it. When you think about all the chemicals and pesticides (as well as all of their harmful effects) that you're avoiding, the improved nutrition you can gain, and the contribution you're making to saving Mother Nature, that extra bit of effort you're taking in adhering to an organic lifestyle doesn't seem like so much anymore, does it?

Chapter 8

Growing Your Own Home Garden

MANY PEOPLE TODAY are turning to a plant-based diet as an alternative to diets too rich in saturated meat products, junk food, and highly processed foods. In some cases, it can involve spending time in the produce section of your local grocery store, looking for fruits and vegetables that are grown organically and spending extra money on them.

You can follow a great plant-based diet in an even better way while growing your fruits and vegetables in your own home garden, and it really isn't all that hard! If you live in an apartment, you can start a container garden in front of a sunny window. If you have a plot of land to turn into a garden, you can go big with a garden filled with healthy fruits and vegetables. You can grow almost anything in a small garden, so you have the spring, summer, and fall to eat off your own land!

Furthermore, small-scale farming and home gardening can have many positive effects on our lives—benefits that range from physical to social to mental. There is nothing so stress-relieving than working an afternoon in your own garden, growing your own healthy foods. In the city, where there is less space for gardening, community gardens have sprung up which bring people together in a positive and enjoyable way.

People can spend more time out in the sun tending their gardens, and this adds to the vitamin D content of our bodies. You can be more physically fit by working in an organic garden. You get to use your muscles on a regular basis, and you will be growing foods that are actually healthy to all parts of our body.

Last, you can feel comfortable that you are not adding to the destruction of the earth and its valuable soil, and putting your hands in the dirt can be soothing and can bring about a greater sense of calm. With the simple act of growing your own garden, you get so many benefits in return!

As mentioned, putting up your own home garden is actually quite simple. You can start with just a few pots and grow your own tomatoes and peppers. If you have the space, though, you might want to start a garden in your yard. If that's the case, here are a few tips to get you started on your very own home garden.

Find the Right Spot

Of course, there are a lot of things to consider when finding the most desirable ground to plant your vegetables. In fact, having the right soil composition matters the most when choosing your garden spot. Healthy soil is essential for growing a healthy garden.

There are various soil test kits that help you determine the pH level of your soil and the type of soil you are dealing with. You would most probably want to plant on loamy soil, as most plants thrive in this type of dirt, and it contains the most nutrients. Determining the pH level of your soil allows you to gauge whether your vegetables get the nutrients they need to grow. An acidic or alkaline soil might impede the absorption of nutrients. The best time to get your soil tested is during spring or fall when it is the most stable.

Find the right area where your plants will receive the most sunlight. Vibrant, lush vegetables require at least six hours of sunlight daily to grow, so make sure your garden isn't shaded with tall trees and other household structures.

Having a water source nearby is important. Your vegetables will require you to water them regularly and properly, so make sure a garden hose is accessible.

Structuring Your Garden

Before you begin planting, have a clear map or plan of whatever part of your garden you intend to grow your vegetables on. Keep in mind that there are certain plants that grow well together, and there are those that do not. More importantly, proper spacing gives you the most out of your garden without compromising your plants' ability to grow.

It is also advisable to plot your garden on paper first and then transfer those plans into reality on your lot. Outlining your lot with strings will help you visualize the spacing and the type of vegetables you intend to plant. Plotting also helps you maximize your garden because you might have to allow too much space for pathways, when some careful planning could have helped you make more efficient use of your space. For a smaller garden, or for those just starting out, it is easier to divide your lot into four parts or quadrants, with each quadrant supporting a certain type of plant. For example, in one quadrant, you can have rows of herbs, and in another, rows of leafy greens. This way, the crops are neatly planted, making it easier to work on them and giving them the right amount of space to grow. Plus, it helps you reach every nook and cranny without stepping on your other crops.

Cultivating, harvesting, replanting, and crop rotating would be a lot easier too.

Many gardeners incorporate flowers into their garden structures. Not only are flowers beautiful to look at, they also attract insects and other organisms that make your garden healthier and more alive.

Make sure to make a planting calendar! Mark the months in which your intended vegetables should grow and mature, and plan your replanting schedules and harvest periods as well. It is also very important to take note of the first frost dates in a year because this is what determines planting periods for most vegetables.

Preparing Your Yard

Once you've gotten everything planned out, clearing the ground is the first step in working your soil. Clear the ground of shrubs and weeds, allowing the soil to be crumbly and loose. Generally, you want the soil to loosen up because compacted ground, especially during winter time, isn't good for your vegetables.

Using organic fertilizer in the form of homemade compost or aged manure will liven up your soil and replenish lost nutrients. Using chemical fertilizers might be easier, but they contain a relatively small amount of nutrients. More importantly, the chemical residue might pollute the soil, the plants, and bodies of water around it.

If you want an especially fruitful garden, consider starting a compost pile or box. All you need to do is put in vegetation and clippings from around your yard, add food scraps and paper, and mix everything with a little bit of soil. Worms thrive in the moist environment of a good compost heap so that you will soon have rich soil that will make your home garden thrive. Adding organic matter also helps the soil retain moisture to allow nutrients to remain in it. With this, you allow the plants and other microorganisms to thrive in your garden. Microorganisms help bind nutrients to the soil for the plants to absorb.

The Organic Option

If you decide to have a backyard home garden, give some thought to if you want to grow organic foods or not. Organic gardening is a great choice because the food is grown without pesticides, herbicides, or fungicides. The natural options cease to become an option and, rather, become mandatory in your garden. This means no harmful chemicals exist with the food you pick, and you can even eat them straight out of the garden without having to wash them extensively.

When you decide to grow organically, you are committing to growing food naturally. This means that instead of chemicals, you use mulch, manure, or compost to fertilize the garden. You are committing to weeding, watering, and harvesting the vegetables and fruits when they become ripe. Since no chemicals are involved in maintaining an organic garden, the food will be free of poisons and much healthier for you than most of the foods you get at the grocery store.

As an up-and-coming organic gardener, you will learn how to grow foods holistically and with health as a priority. Your own grown vegetables and fruits will contain valuable nutrients, such as vitamins, minerals, and antioxidants for better health. These foods haven't yet had these nutrients leached from the long packing and delivery process. You simply go out your door and pick them at their peak of freshness.

As an organic gardener, you might also have to learn about crop rotation. As mentioned above, this is when you grow one type of food for one year in a single place and alternate it with another food the next season or year, and this option requires prior planning. This is because different foods take and give back to the soil in differing amounts, and you can use some nutrients from the food you grew the season or year before to nourish the food you are growing now.

In addition, a compost pile, as mentioned earlier, becomes a vital component of your gardening system. No longer will you throw your meal scraps away, but instead, you will keep them in a compost heap that is regularly turned and aerated with a pitchfork. Worms in the compost heap then convert raw matter into healthy black dirt. The compost pile, which can contain leaves, dirt, food remains, and manure that all mix together, ensures that you have the best soil and fertilizer available and allows you to stay away from store-bought and potentially unnatural fertilizers that cost additional money.

There are numerous guides online for organic vegetable gardening, as well as many books on the topic. In reality, though, the best teacher is experience, so learn the initial steps, get the supplies, and just do it!

In the meantime, if you're looking for good crops to start with, jump to the next chapters for some great suggestions!

Chapter 9

Great Crops to Plant in Your Home Garden

So you've decided that having your own home garden is right for you in your vegan journey, have you? If you're not sure what to plant and where, then you've come to the right place! In this chapter, we'll discuss some common crops in home gardening. I'll let you know about their nutritional properties, so you know why they're worth having in your garden, as well as offer you some quick tips on planting and growing them yourself.

Tomatoes

Tomatoes lend themselves well to container gardening and can even grow like wild in the good earth of your backyard. They are also one of the most versatile foods that you can plant in your backyard. Use them for sandwiches, salads, snacks, fresh sauces, and even for juicing. With their sweet, and sometimes tangy, flavor, salsa, sauces and salads become more flavorful with just a handful of slices.

People often mistake tomatoes as vegetables, but tomatoes are actually fruits which are part of the nightshade family, related to chilies and peppers. The different varieties of tomatoes are perfect for creating tasty dishes in an array of cooking styles and flavor profiles.

Cherry tomatoes are among the sweetest kinds, usually thrown in with leafy vegetables for quick salads.

The distinct tomato red color is actually from the lycopene, a phytochemical that's packed in many fruits. Lycopene is known to have antioxidant properties that fight off free radicals in the body, destroying them before they attach to our cells and cause diseases. It is also believed to prevent certain kinds of cancer, reduce the bad cholesterol in the bloodstream, and lower blood pressure levels.

Tomatoes are usually planted indoors away from the frosty soils from February to April. Transplant them outdoors when the soil is warm, either into a pot tilled with compost or directly into the ground. Make sure the plant is regularly watered and is receiving enough sunlight. When the fruit is ripe and brightly colored by July, it's good to go.

Onions

Onions are related to scallions, chives, leeks, and garlic and are of the *allium* family of vegetables. They have been grown in gardens for many centuries where they have been used both for medicinal properties and for cooking.

Onions are such a perfect addition to so many dishes that it's always a great idea to have some of them ready in your home at all times. They keep for several weeks before sprouting and have numerous health benefits. For home gardeners, the best part about onions is that they are easy to grow and can be used over a long period if stored in a cool dry place. You can grow a nice row of them in your garden, harvesting them either as they develop or all at once—depending on your needs.

Onions are also very versatile. They can have a somewhat sweet flavor or can have a spicy, pungent, and sharp flavor, depending on what variety of onions you use, and on when you harvest them in the year. As a rule of thumb, young onions tend to be sweeter, so if that's how you like your onions, try to go for the youngest ones you can find.

Because onions are so ubiquitous in cooking, it's easy to over-look the fact that they have so many health benefits and medicinal properties. Here are some of the great health benefits that come with eating onions:

- For those who want to trim down the pounds, onions are low in calories and contain no fat or cholesterol, meaning they're a great choice to help fill you up without leaving you hungry and unsatisfied.
- They also happen to be rich in fiber, which can help with digestion and the smoother passage of stool.
- Onions each contain about fifteen grams of plant carbohy-drates and no raw sugar.
- Onions are known to help reduce the risk of heart disease, diabetes, and metabolic syndrome.
- Onions contain several kinds of minerals, including iron, folic acid, calcium, phosphorus, potassium, and magnesium.
- Onions reduce the risk of colon and rectal cancers. This is because onions contain organosulfur components that inhibit cancer in multiple ways. First, as potent antioxi-dants, organosulfurs help prevent oxygen-free radical formation. These free radicals damage the cells, and can eventually lead to cancer. In addition, organosulfurs also directly block the growth of tumors and can prevent nor-mal cells from mutating into cancer cells.
- Onions are also rich in vitamin C, another excellent anti-oxidant. Skin and other tissues that rely on the presence of healthy collagen also need vitamin C.
- Onions can also be beneficial to your mood and sleep-ing habits. Onions are rich in folic acid, which is known to reduce the risk of depression in humans by decreasing homocysteine levels in the body. Too much homocysteine is known to conflict with the making of serotonin, norepi-nephrine, and dopamine, all of which are essential neuro-chemicals for depression prevention.

Peas and Beans

Peas and beans can also grow in containers or in your backyard garden. They are rich in phytonutrients and have their maximum potency if you simply pick what you need and eat them as soon as possible. In fact, you get the greatest amount of healthy phytonutrients and antioxidants in the food shortly after picking them.

Peas and beans are part of the legume family, together with lentils and chickpeas and twenty other species. Legumes are distinct plants that bear fleshy seeds in an enclosed pod, and are usually purchased canned or dried. Growing your own legume varieties, however, allows you to make fresh hummus, stews, and purees that are all full of protein, vitamin B, and fiber.

Legumes are also perfect for replenishing the lost nutrients in the soil. Typically, planting the same kind of plant over and over again in one patch of soil may mean using up the same nutrients in the soil every time. Planting legumes helps nitrogen-fixing bacteria in the soil to feed the legumes with nutrients while, at the same time, incorporating nitrogen back to the soil. Nitrogen helps plants grow and function properly, which is why it's the most common ingredient in most fertilizers.

Lima Beans

Lima beans are easy to grow in your own garden; they provide an excellent source of many different nutrients and can be used in a variety of recipes. They are a starchy vegetable and are sometimes known as butter beans because of their smooth, buttery texture. Fresh lima beans are usually hard to find, and you can buy them dried or canned. As such, they make a great addition to any home garden, as through your own efforts, you'll have access to those hard-to-find fresh lima beans when they ripen in the late summer and autumn.

Lima beans grow looking like a regular green bean, although the pods are flatter than regular beans. Lima beans need to be shucked out of the pods, with each pod yielding two to four fresh lima beans. Lima beans are usually green or cream-colored, but there are other varieties that come in different colors, including red, purple, black, brown, and white.

Like many other foods you'll be growing, lima beans provide the most nutrition when they are picked fresh from the garden and are cooked and eaten right away. You can eat them alone, salted, or incorporate them into soups and casseroles. When cooled, cooked lima beans also make an excellent addition to green salads. If you want to have your lima beans at their healthiest, try soaking the dried beans in water and cook them without salt, only adding the salt after cooking.

If you want to learn more about the health benefits of lima beans, here are some nutritional facts about them:

- Lima beans are a type of legume, which means they are an excellent source of fiber.
- Because lima beans are rich in insoluble fiber, they can help bulk up your stool and allow for more regular bowel movements and less constipation. This makes them amazing for people who have digestive tract problems, such as diverticulitis and irritable bowel syndrome.
- As mentioned, the high-fiber content of lima beans means they can help those with high cholesterol and diabetes. Lima beans have a low glycemic index and soluble fiber, which is the type of fiber used in binding cholesterol. Fiber also binds with the bile acids in the duodenum. It is bile acids that go on in the metabolic process to make cholesterol, which puts you at risk for heart disease. Thanks to fiber, bile acids instead pass right through the digestive system without being absorbed and made into cholesterol.
- The low glycemic index of lima beans, meanwhile, means that it doesn't allow for a rush of glucose into the system after eating them, meaning the pancreas doesn't get over-stressed, and blood sugar is kept in check and stays level.
- Lima beans have been extensively studied as sources of heart disease protection. One study looked at over sixteen thousand men across the world who were at risk of

heart disease by virtue of being middle-aged men. The study found that those men who ate more legumes had a decreased risk of heart disease over the twenty-five-year period that the study was conducted. Another study looked at men eating high-fiber foods, including lima beans, in the United States. Of these adults who were followed for more than nineteen years, those who ate twenty-one grams of fiber per day had a 12 percent smaller chance of coming down with heart disease as compared to the people who ate less than five grams of fiber per day. The water-soluble fiber was determined to serve as one of the best protections against heart disease.

- Lima beans contain high amounts of magnesium and folate per serving. Folate is a vitamin that lowers the quantity of homocysteine in the bloodstream, which is a risk factor for all forms of heart disease, including stroke, heart attack, and peripheral vascular disease. The magnesium in lima beans, meanwhile, acts as calcium channel blockers, which lowers blood pressure and improves the flow of nutrients and oxygen within the bloodstream. A lack of magnesium in the diet can lead to heart attacks and the liberation of oxygen-free radicals in the body, which is dangerous to the cells of the body.

- Lima beans are a great healthy source of iron too, since just a cup can already contain around a quarter of the daily recommended value of iron. Since they are low in calories and pretty much fat-free, they can help make sure that you never have to turn back to meat for your iron needs.

Soybeans

These days, people can consume in soybeans in many ways. Most people enjoy soybeans after they have been processed in a factory to make soymilk, soy flour, miso, tofu, and tempeh. While ready-made sources of soybeans are very widely available for purchase, an even better option would be to grow them yourself in your garden or field, harvest them, and cook them up in various dishes.

Soybeans are high in protein, which makes them an excellent protein source for vegans who need nonmeat sources of protein. Soybeans are a source of complete proteins and have the best nutrients when you harvest them from your own garden and cook them fresh. They can be used in a very wide variety of dishes, which is great news for home garden owners. Furthermore, soy protein is particularly helpful in that it contains eight essential amino acids, which cannot be synthesized by the body.

There are many guides to growing soybeans, but generally, they need about three months of warm weather to mature. You can get various varieties of seeds to plant, but all of them need nitrogen-fixing bacteria, and there are products available specifically for soybean plants. The proper bacterium helps the beans to absorb nitrogen from the air and store it in their root nodules, which aids the growth of the plant, helps in bean production and improves soil fertility. To make the best use of the soybeans you grow in your own garden, pick them when they are green and boil them until soft.

If you're still not convinced about how valuable soybeans can be to you as a home gardener, here are a few more reasons to help you out:

- Soybeans contain 43 percent total protein, which is twice as much as other legumes. The protein quality in soybeans is the best you'll find, with the highest rating of food proteins as defined by the World Health Organization and the US FDA.
- Unlike many plants that contain incomplete proteins, soybeans are a complete protein source. This means it contains all the essential amino acids for life, including those that can't be individually synthesized by the body. In fact, it has the same quality of protein as is found in milk and other meat sources, but with a lot less fat.
- Soybeans contain about 19 percent healthy fat, which is more than most legumes other than peanuts. While fat

is often referred to as a bad thing in your diet, plant fats are actually essential for a healthy diet. Plant fats contain essential fatty acids that can't be directly made within the body, but which are necessary for the synthesis of cell membranes and other cellular structures. Plant-based fat found in soybeans is usually of the unsaturated type, which means it is a particularly beneficial fat, although there are some monounsaturated and saturated fats in soybeans (about 14 percent of total fat).

- Soybeans contain omega 3 fatty acids, which are known to be protective against both cancer and heart disease. Besides this, linolenic acid is another of the healthy fats found in soybeans; it has direct protective effects on the body's health. You can choose to eat a lot of soybean fat in soybean oil or just a little fat in soybean flour, which has almost all the soybean oil removed during processing. You can also eat reduced-fat sources of soybeans, including low-fat tofu and nonfat soymilk.

- A single serving of soybeans contains about eight grams of healthy fiber. This is best obtained when you pick and cook your own soybeans in dishes at home. Soymilk and tofu alone have had much of their fiber removed in the processing of these foods, while tempeh, textured soy protein, and soy flour are high in fiber.

- Soybeans and foods containing soybeans are rich in calcium. Tofu alone has about 120–750 mg of calcium in just a half-cup serving. You can get up to a 100 mg of calcium per cup of soymilk, and if you purchase naturally calcium-fortified soymilk, you can get two to three times that much calcium per cup.

- Soybean-based milk is also a good source of vitamin D, which, as you might recall, helps the body in the absorption of calcium. Because of this, the calcium found in soymilk is absorbed well in the digestive system—about as well as the body's absorption rate of calcium in milk.

- Fermented foods that contain or are made out of soybeans, such as miso and tempeh, contain a lot of absorbable iron, which helps in the production of the red blood cells that carry oxygen all over our bodies.
- For those who are worried about their vitamin B12 intake, all soybean-created foods are high in B complex vitamins, and soymilk is also usually fortified with healthy vitamin B12.

Radishes

Radishes take only a few weeks to become edible, and after pulling them up, you instantly have room to grow a row of something else. They mature very quickly and take up very little space, making radishes one of the most common salad staples in everyone's home garden.

Varieties of radishes are usually characterized depending on their seasonality. European varieties are generally planted in cooler spring weather and are usually smaller. The Japanese name *daikon* has been used to refer to all Asian varieties that are white-skinned and longer in length, so when you hear the term daikon, it might not actually be referring to just a single variant, but to a bunch of similar radish variants that grow in Asia.

Radishes are a good source of vitamin C, which makes them good for boosting your immune system to fight off disease and for helping create collagen in your body, which strengthens your blood vessel walls. Radishes are also considered to be roughage, or indigestible starches, that can facilitate the body's water retention, promote digestive health, and give you the feeling of being full for hours. As a natural diuretic, radishes help heal urinary pains and inflammation too.

Carrots

Carrots are among the most favored root vegetables out there. This is in part due to their versatility. They can be used as a snack on their own or as a texture enhancer in many salads. They can be cooked or taken raw, and whatever way you have them, they're sure to make your meal more interesting.

Carrots belong to the same botanical family as parsley, dill, and celery. Carrots grow best in sandy soil or in very loose, rock-free soil. When harvesting, make sure to not bruise the roots and to handpick them.

Most people are highly familiar with orange carrots, but carrots actually come in a number of varieties, some of which have white, purple, and even reddish hues. Regardless of the color, carrots are an excellent source of beta-carotene. Our livers convert beta-carotene to vitamin A, which in turn helps the retinas of the eyes manufacture necessary compounds for better vision, especially at night. Vitamin A also is linked to decreasing the risk of eyesight degeneration and cataracts. Beta-carotene acts as an antioxidant, which slows the aging process and all the diseases that result from aging.

Potatoes

Potatoes are among the most widely produced type of crop, owing to their versatility as an ingredient and their nutritional value. It's one of those foods that can stand on its own or, as a side, can be prepared in a variety of ways and can really help make any event or occasion become more interesting.

Potatoes are part of the Solanaceae family, together with tomatoes, squash, and eggplant. The tuber underground is the edible part of the plant, and it comes in different shapes, colors, and flavors.

Potatoes are fairly easy to sow and take care of. In fact, there is a growing trend of gardeners using black trash bags to grow their tubers. The bags are filled with soil in an upright position, and holes are punched so that the water drains out. Of course, it isn't as aesthetically appealing as you might want it to be, but once the tubers have grown, it is easier to empty the bags and collect the potatoes instead of digging them up one by one. Also, because the bags are black, they absorb more heat from the sun, thus speeding up the early stages of the growing process.

It is important to keep in mind that planting potatoes in areas that have been previously planted with other members of the Solanaceae should be avoided, as it makes the potatoes more vulnerable to blight.

Squash

Both potatoes and squash need the entire summer to become available for eating and are relatively low-maintenance, so all you really need to do is to keep them weed-free and watch them grow. In the early autumn or late summer, you can dig up the potatoes and harvest the squash. What's more, these types of produce can be kept at room temperature or in a cool place for many months, so you have instant winter eating from vegetables you grew in the summer.

Squash belongs to a family of plants called Cucurbitaceae and is related to melons, watermelons, and cucumbers. Varieties of squash are usually divided into two main types: winter and summer squash. Winter squash generally refers to those varieties that can be stored until December. They generally have an orange or deeper yellow color and are the most common varieties around. Butternut, banana, acorn, and pumpkin squash are all winter squashes. Varieties of summer squash mature quickly and are marketable all year round.

As vine-type plants, winter squash varieties tend to use up a lot of garden space, but they can be planted directly inground or on garden hill beds. It is recommended to warm the soil with mulch or wait till midsummer to prevent plant diseases and pests. Pay attention to your fruits as they grow; misshapen fruits may be the result of inadequate or irregular watering.

Of course, at this point, some of us might be thinking, "So what's the difference between a pumpkin and a squash?" I know I wasn't sure when I started off as a vegan, but the answer's actually pretty simple: a pumpkin is a type of squash. Also, pumpkin seeds are edible, unlike other squash varieties. If you want to get more out of the area of your garden devoted to squash, then consider planting pumpkins, so you can make use of the seeds as a snack. Also, it's pretty awesome having your own personal source for pumpkins when Halloween swings by!

Kale

Many call kale a superfood, and for good reason. Kale is one of the most in demand varieties of leafy greens for its exceptional nutritional value and medicinal properties. It is one of the most nutrient-dense foods that anyone can find, so having it in our backyards and free from fertilizer residue is one thing we can all benefit from.

Kale belongs to the Brassica family of plants, together with cabbage, cauliflower, broccoli, and Brussels sprouts. Several varieties are available, including the ornamental, curly, and dinosaur, and all differ in texture and taste.

Most leafy greens are high in flavonoids—nutrient groups that exhibit antioxidant properties. For kale, in particular, there is a huge array of powerful flavonoids—such as quercetin and kaempferol, to name a few—that counteract aging and cancer-causing free radicals in the body. Kale has also a large concentration of beta-carotene, which is linked to a decrease in the risk of cancerous cell formations and obstructive heart diseases.

Research has shown that eating kale lowers the risk of cardiovascular diseases in the long-term because it lowers the overall cholesterol levels in the body. Essentially, compounds in kale bind with the bile acids produced in the liver and help flush them out of the body instead of reusing them and injecting them into the bloodstream. Some researchers even believe that steamed kale is half as potent as cholesterol-lowering drugs in the market.

Kale may be the greatest source of vitamin K; a cup of steamed kale has at least five times the recommended daily intake of vitamin K. Vitamin K helps regulate blood clotting, circulation, and the body's inflammatory processes. It also helps increase bone density and decrease instances of bone fracture and loss for women undergoing the menopausal stage.

Kale is fairly easy to grow and can be harvested all-winter with very minimal care. Mulching the ground helps warm the soil and improve yields.

Lettuce and Salad Greens

Lettuce and other greens can be grown and harvested all summer long for salads that are high in phytonutrients and antioxidants. All you need to do is harvest some of the leaves, wash them, and toss them together for a healthy salad that can come with tomatoes, carrots, or radishes that you also grew yourself. This is the core of a plant-based diet that will give you benefits far beyond a meat-based diet.

Salad greens are practically the base or the bed of every salad. They are usually served raw and are tossed with other ingredients with a light dressing. A good salad is a balanced salad, so having something sweet like fruits, and/or something salty and crunchy makes any salad green more enjoyable to eat. Lettuce and its varieties are the most common salad beds, but there are other varieties that you need to be familiar with.

Lettuce

This low-calorie green contains phytonutrients that have disease prevention properties. Aside from filling you up, lettuce also contains vitamin A and beta-carotene, vitamin K, and folic acid.

Lettuce is one of those sturdy plants that can tolerate shade. It matures fastest with sun and can be planted in container or pots. In fact, some people find it more desirable to plant lettuce beside taller plants like tomatoes to save more space and for a more aesthetically appealing garden.

Lettuces are grouped into these four varieties:

1. Crisp head

Iceberg lettuce or crisp head lettuce tend to form rounder, more tightly-packed heads. They have paler green leaves and are more valued for their crunch. Crisp head lettuce is usually eaten cold with heavier dressings or paired with more flavorful ingredients.

2.   Looseleaf

Compared to the crisp head, looseleaf doesn't form a round, compact head. Instead, the leaves are more scattered, larger, and curlier. The leaves are also arranged in a short, central stalk that can be pulled. This variety has a mild sweet taste and is usually used in sandwiches and hors d'oeuvres.

3.   Butterhead

The leaves of this variety are tender and mild, hence the name butterhead. They form loosely around a round head and have a smoother texture to them. As delicate as they are, they make simple plates look great.

4.   Romaine

Perhaps one of the more popular kinds of lettuce, romaine has longer leaves and is the traditional green used in the popular Caesar salad. The outer leaves are darker in color and sometimes more bitter. Romaine can also be used as sandwich wrappers and bring a satisfying texture to wonderful salads.

Salad Greens

Belgian Endive

Due to their shape, Belgian endives serve as elegant "spoons" in salad beds. They have a slightly bitter taste. Part of the chicory family (together with other salad greens: escarole, frisee, and chicory), they mesh well with creamy dressings. They are usually grown underground but maintain their delicate, pale color. Belgian endive thrives in cooler temperatures, even up to a light ground frost.

Radicchio

This vibrantly colored plant isn't necessarily green in color, but it is used in many salads. Once cooked, the usual bitter taste turns into a delicate, sweet flavor. This plant has different varieties, each named after the places in the Veneto region of Italy from which they are found. Some varieties tend to be rounder, while others have flatter, broader leaves like the rest of the plants in the same family. It is also a cool-weather crop that's grown alongside cabbage and cauliflower. Set plants in the garden during spring and make sure the soil maintains moisture as the head begins to grow.

Spinach

Spinach, like kale, is densely packed with nutrients which makes it a great salad green as well as a delicious side. It is an excellent source of antioxidant nutrients—vitamin C, vitamin E, and carotenoids—that fight diseases and early signs of aging. Researchers have also found that age-related vision impairments can be improved by the antioxidant properties of spinach. The vitamin K in this green also helps promote better bone health. Although it tends to be sandy; washing spinach lends it ready to be served and prepared.

Watercress

Don't be fooled by its tiny leaves—watercress has that peppery, tangy flavor that can give any salad a kick. Rich in vitamins C and A, it provides contrast to fruity, sweet salads. Finding the right spot to plant watercress might be tricky though, as it requires a stream or a wet area.

However, you can make your own garden stream with peat moss, small rocks, and a garden hose to allow this tasty plant to grow.

Arugula

Like other greens, arugula is a low-calorie vegetable that's rich in antioxidants, folates, and phytochemicals. The younger leaves tend to have a milder, sweeter taste than the mature ones do. But with balsamic vinegar dressing, this green can be used as an herb to flavor salads or be eaten like spinach. Growing arugula is fairly simple, as they grow rapidly and can be planted for early spring and fall time harvest.

Microgreens

Don't confuse microgreens with sprouts; microgreens are harvested, or cut, earlier while they are smaller in size and less mature. The increasing use of microgreens in salads and as a garnish is largely because of the intense flavor they can provide as well as their dense nutritional content. And you don't really need a spot in your garden to grow them; microgreens grow best in seedling trays right beside your windowsill.

Organic Sprouts

Sprouts are very young shoots of plants such as alfalfa, sunflower, or soybean that are eaten as raw vegetables. Because they are essentially regular plants that are taken early in their life cycles, sprouts are some of the healthiest plant food sources. They are extremely nutrient-dense superfoods that can easily boost your nutrient intake.

There are simply loads of reasons to grow and consume your own sprouts. They can contain live micronutrients that improve their nutritional value, can have as much as one hundred more natural enzymes than most raw fruits and vegetables and can also contain large amounts of antioxidants. They are rich sources of energy and vitamins (especially when consumed fresh, raw, and young). In addition, sprouts contain plenty of vegetable protein (which helps many different cellular processes), have a lot of healthy fiber for your digestive tract and contain magnesium, calcium, and essential fatty acids.

These leafy vegetables are a great, inexpensive food that can be used in many dishes to make your meal healthier. Put them in your salads, sandwiches, wraps, or just about any dish, and enjoy the healthful punch that even just a small amount can pack!

Not all sprouts are created alike, however, and each kind of sprout has its own brand of nutritional qualities. So it pays to have a nice variety of them growing in your home garden. Here are some vegetable sprouts that provide distinct nutritional benefits:

- *Broccoli sprouts.* These sprouts have high amounts of healthy phytochemicals, including the precursor molecule to sulforaphane, an essential part of good nutrition.
- *Alfalfa sprouts.* These contain a lot of healthy phytoestrogens and other phytochemicals. They are high in saponins and canavanine, as well as good sources of vitamins A, B, C, D, E, and K.
- *Lentil sprouts.* Lentils are high in protein, with a protein content of about 26 percent. They can be eaten raw like any other sprout.
- *Clover sprouts.* These contain a great deal of phytochemicals and isoflavones.
- *Mung bean sprouts.* They are a great source of plant protein and a good source of vitamins A and C.
- *Sunflower sprouts.* These are rich in essential fatty acids, as well as other types of healthy fats, fiber, minerals, and phytosterols. They are high in protein and contain many vitamins.
- *Pea shoot sprouts.* Pea shoots are an excellent source of folic acid, vitamin A, vitamin C, magnesium, and zinc. They are a good source of protein as well.

Chapter 10

Great Health-Promoting Herbs You Can Grow at Home

As HAS BEEN made abundantly clear in this book, plant foods are some of the best sources of vital nutrition. Of these plant foods, herbs can provide a plethora of health benefits and add low-calorie flavor to a variety of dishes. Furthermore, herbs can also be used medicinally as all-natural and very cheap remedies to common minor injuries. In fact, some herbs have been found through research or through traditional Chinese medicine to help people stay healthy through the plant phytochemicals they contain.

If you're starting your own home garden, herbs are a great choice, as they tend to be easy to grow and are dense in nutrients. Here are five of the best health-promoting herbs that you can grow at home.

Echinacea

Echinacea is also called the purple coneflower and it grows from one to two feet tall in your garden or around your house. It was used in ancient cultures as a way of reducing many of the symptoms of viral infections, such as the cold or flu and other infectious illnesses. It is also available at health food stores and some pharmacies in pill or tincture form. You can make a tea of the echinacea plant whenever you feel a cold coming on.

Echinacea contains many valuable substances for your health. These include phenols, which are strong antioxidants and which regulate certain enzymes and human cell receptors in the human body. These herbs also have alkylamides, which directly affect your immune system when faced with an infection.

Basil

Basil is an annual herb that is especially perfect for container gardens. All you need to do is harvest the leaves and stems of the herb. Basil flavors many different dishes. Pesto sauce is made with fresh basil and garlic and contains a wide variety of healthy nutrients. Try to harvest the youngest leaves as soon as possible. Besides being delicious, basil can help improve your appetite, control flatulence, and improve healing of cuts or scrapes.

Chamomile

This plant grows as a white daisy-like flower and is best grown near the house where you have ready access to it. The heads of the flowers are used for their health benefits, including the management of colic, indigestion, skin irritations, inflammations, and anxiety. Chamomile can be infused in a tea form or worked into a salve that can be directly applied to the skin for better health.

Feverfew

Feverfew is best grown in flower gardens because they make nice white daisy-like flowers. Both the leaves and flowers of this healthful herb can be brewed into a tea or chewed directly for the relief of various kinds of headaches, as well as arthritis, pain, and various skin conditions. It can also be made into a salve so that it can be directly applied to the affected skin.

Lavender

You can incorporate this herb into your flower garden, as it makes lovely purple flowers. It is used as an essential oil for aromatherapy. It is said that to smell lavender is relaxing and calming to both the mind and body. Lavender is also a great pain reliever and can be directly applied or incorporated into a salve in order to apply it to bruises and cuts. It acts like an antiseptic herb when applied to affected areas of the skin.

The benefits of many of these herbs are that they are beautiful in your garden and can be picked fresh for the best potency of their active ingredients. Some can even be grown in a pot in your house to be placed in front of a sunny window.

Some of the herbs will be perennials, meaning that they will pop up every year in the same place without the need for replanting. Others are annual plants so once they have been picked, you need to lay down some seed to grow some more.

However, which way you choose to plant them, home-grown herbs are always a great addition to a healthy vegan lifestyle!

Chapter 11

The Raw Diet And Its Many Benefits

How To Get Started On A Raw Food Diet

IF YOU'RE SERIOUS about changing your lifestyle and overcoming tinnitus, you'll want to start incorporating more fresh produce, nuts, and other uncooked fare into your regular routine. Though a raw food diet isn't difficult per se, it does require a good deal of planning. Besides speaking to your doctor or healthcare professional, you'll want to spend time preparing your body for some of the changes it will encounter as it adapts to your new eating habits.

A raw food diet is defined as one in which 70-90% of all calories come from uncooked foods. Most people understand this to mean uncooked produce; however, there are those who will also consume raw eggs, dairy, and meat. I myself though am a vegetarian, and so I can only speak of my own experiences and my own methods to cure tinnitus.

You'll want to devote a reasonable amount of time to planning new meals given the limitations of the raw food diet. Simply because you're choosing to eat food in its natural state though doesn't mean your meals have to be bland. You can transform a plate of raw veggies by slicing, dicing, chopping, and even blending them. Salad bars have become increasingly popular, and if you're creative with your choice of dressing, you can create a truly satisfying meal. Many raw eaters also consume their calories as smoothies because as long as you don't heat the food above 112°F, you'll still get all of the same nutrients.

Most people who attempt the raw food diet introduce raw food little by little. However, be careful not to mix raw and cooked foods in one meal. When combined, cooked foods will neutralize many of the enzymes and nutrients present in the raw food thereby defeating the entire purpose of the diet. Mixing cooked and raw food also forces the digestive system to work harder than it needs to. Instead, decide to designate a meal or snack every day as a raw meal and gradually increase the amount of raw food you eat each day as well as the frequency in which you eat it.

If you've eaten primarily cooked and processed foods your whole life, the raw food diet can really shock your system especially if it's a long-term plan. Raw food diets are usually deficient in iron, zinc, vitamin D, vitamin B12, and omega-3 fatty acids. Because these vitamins are derived primarily from animal sources, vegans and vegetarians tend to suffer to an even greater extent.

A raw food diet is designed to cleanse toxins from your body, and so you should expect some discomfort. Cravings for sugar and salt especially over the first several days are fairly normal and should eventually subside. However, if you start experiencing prolonged headaches, nausea, or mild depression, you should consider supplementing your diet with fortified grains or multi-vitamins to accommodate your body's needs.

The raw food diet isn't always easy, but if you plan your meals ahead of time and monitor your body's reactions carefully, you will set yourself up for success. Though raw food on its own won't necessarily cure your tinnitus, it can ultimately help rid your body of harmful toxins and provide it with the enzymes it needs to help your body function normally.

Taking Proper Precautions

A raw food diet affords its followers countless benefits, but the diet may not be for everyone. Even those with tinnitus should exercise caution before beginning such a restrictive diet because you may in fact be cutting yourself off from many of the nutrients your body desperately needs.

Before changing your diet completely, you should take your own nutritional requirements into account. Then make sure to speak with your family practitioner to ask whether you're healthy enough to start a raw-food diet. That being said, the raw food diet need not be more difficult than necessary if you're armed with the proper tools and strategies for success.

Children:

Even if the raw food diet works for you, it may not work for your kids. Children are growing at a rapid rate, and their bodies and, perhaps even more importantly, their brains need more nutrients per pound of body weight than adults to develop normally.

Malnutrition is a very real and potent threat for pre-pubescent children and failing to provide them with the vitamins and minerals they need may result in severe mental and physical disabilities later on in life. If you want to place your children on a partially raw diet, do so with extreme caution and make sure to discuss any changes with their pediatrician.

Pregnant & Nursing Women

So too, pregnant and nursing women should steer clear of raw food diets for the sake of their children or future children. The food the mother eats will directly affect the health of the child, and so you should go to extra lengths to eat a well-rounded diet. Your daily intake of protein and calcium will increase substantially, and it's extremely difficult to fulfill all of your needs on a raw diet.

Even if you choose to cut back on cooked foods when your child is older, you should temporarily avoid any restrictive or extreme diets. Remember you're nourishing a developing life, and the decisions you make during this time period could have very serious consequences.

Diseases & Disorders

Certain disorders and diseases require you to take in more of a specific kind of nutrient to compensate for any shortages. Your body needs calcium to build strong bones especially if you have osteoporosis. Women ages 51 and older should be taking 1,200mg of calcium every day at the very least, and since the body doesn't produce its own calcium, you have to get it through the foods you eat.

You can get calcium through leafy greens, but many still come up short. While you can buy oatmeal and breakfast cereals that have been fortified with calcium, it's preferable to rely on natural sources of the mineral.

Anemia, a condition caused by either a lack of red blood cells or a lack of hemoglobin, the protein that binds oxygen, is a relatively common condition that results in fatigue, shortness of breath, dizziness, and insomnia. It's particularly common among pregnant women, young children, and the elderly. However, it can be easily treated with iron.

Though your doctor may prescribe iron supplements for anemia, you'll aggravate the condition further if you rely solely on these vitamins. The top sources of iron happen to come from mostly animal sources. Vegetables also contains iron, but you'd have to eat a cup of cooked beans, for example, to get the same amount of iron you'd get from only 3oz. of beef liver or oysters.

Nutrient Deficiencies:

As we've mentioned before, the raw food diet does not provide an adequate amount of every nutrient. If you decide to try cutting out cooked food, you risk eliminating the following nutrients from your diet: iron, calcium, vitamin B-12, vitamin-D, zinc, omega-3 fatty acids, and protein. While you can find calcium, for instance, in some leafy greens, these vitamins are primarily found in animal products.

Deficiencies in these major nutrients can cause severe issues, and it's imperative that you monitor your body's reactions and supplement your diet with vitamins when necessary. If you're only going on the diet temporarily as a way to address some of your tinnitus symptoms, then you may not have to take too many precautions. However, if you plan to implement these health changes over the long-term, you should be in close communication with a general doctor or a nutritionist.

Meal-Planning:

It seems like veganism and other similar diets have developed a negative reputation for themselves, but they're not nearly as expensive as they may seem. In fact, you'll probably save money if you're not purchasing steak, poultry, or fresh fish on a regular basis. Try shopping at your local farmer's market for good deals and remember to shop for food that's fresh and in season. Otherwise, you can always find inexpensive bags of vegetables in the frozen section of your supermarket.

Raw Food Restaurants:

Just because you're beginning a restrictive diet doesn't mean that you'll have to eat every meal at home. This couldn't be further from the truth. Raw food restaurants are popping up in big cities like Chicago, L.A., and New York, and more and more establishments are adding raw food options to their menus.

You'll can also find a range of cafes and restaurants across the country that have expanded their salad bars and transformed simple plates of lettuce into gourmet meals. Never fear that you'll have to sit out on family gatherings and joyous occasions because of your diet.

Making major changes in your daily routine can be stressful, but if you prep properly, eating a raw diet doesn't have to be. Take some time to develop some new recipes and explore some of the food establishments in your local community to see how you can make the raw food diet a reality in your own life.

Debunking Raw Food Diet Myths

As of late, the Raw Food Diet has gained a reputation that has taken it from a diet to a popular lifestyle choice. Celebrities such as Demi Moore, Robin Williams and Alicia Silverstone swear by the raw food diet, and every day more and more celebrities are joining the ranks. There's an entire list of public figures who believe that eating a diet rich in raw fruits and vegetables is the healthiest way to live.

There are those people, however, who shy away from the diet under the assumption that it is inconvenient, expensive, and unhealthy. There are many myths claiming what the Raw Food Diet is and what it isn't. By separating myth from fact, you will be able to properly assess and understand the benefits and drawbacks of the Raw Food diet. Only then you will be able to decide for yourself whether it is the right lifestyle change for you.

Let's talk about what the Raw Food diet is NOT.

The Raw Food diet is not a diet consisting of 100% raw foods alone. For a person to reap the benefits of raw food eating, 2/3 of their diet should come from raw foods. That doesn't mean that you are forbidden from eat foods that are cooked or heated. On the contrary. In certain cases, heating foods actually makes some nutrients more available. It also doesn't mean that you can't deviate from the diet every once in a while. Of course, as with any routine, you won't derive many of the health benefits without dedication and discipline. However, any amount of raw food will be beneficial.

The Raw Food diet is also NOT an expensive diet. It's true that it seems as though lately, diets that are easy on the body are not so easy on our wallets. One only needs to take a look at the Atkins diet, the South Beach diet, Nutrisystem, Jenny Craig, diet pills, drugs, juices…the list goes on and on. But think about it: a diet consisting of mostly raw fruits, vegetables, seeds, sprouts, grains, seaweed, nuts and other cold-pressed raw oils and fermented sauces is not only good for your stomach, but also costs very little. A raw food diet means that you spend your fast food money—the money that you would have spent on that cholesterol-ridden, high-fat cheese-burger—on a healthful salad, packed with nutrients that can help your body release toxins, keep you stay trim, and ultimately improve the quality of your life.

Finally, the Raw Food diet is NOT a boring diet, meaning there is no variety. Like every lifestyle change you make, your success depends on your mentality. You wouldn't decide to go green without first researching what the lifestyle entailed. Likewise, you wouldn't decide to entirely change your eating habits without learning about how to do it properly. When you research the Raw Food diet, you will find that there are hundreds and hundreds of recipes, meal plans, and methods of preparation that make meals not only palatable but delicious and varied. Education, research and a positive, open mind-set make all of the difference in the way that you approach any new lifestyle.

Debunking some of the myths regarding this increasingly pop-ular raw food lifestyle is the first step in educating yourself and ulti-mately deciding whether the Raw Food life is the right choice for you.

The remedies I've developed for tinnitus are designed to give your body the tools it needs to heal itself naturally. Though eating a diet full of produce and fresh fish and meats will fuel your body and brain, you may not be consuming enough vitamins and minerals if the majority of the food you eat is cooked.

Our prehistoric ancestors discovered thousands of years ago that it was far easier to digest food, and in this case meat in particular, if it were cooked first. While produce, and even meat, contain more vitamins and minerals when raw, the body can digest the food better if the food is cooked.

In fact, many argue that the development of culinary arts was an important evolutionary step in human development because it allowed us to absorb nutrients quickly and safely than we were when we were eating raw meat.

Heat partially breaks down a food's protein structure making it more palatable. However, it also partially denatures enzymes and destroys the vitamins meant to aid digestion and fight diseases, like tinnitus.

Though I don't by any means advocate eating uncooked meat like our prehistoric ancestors did, raw fruits and vegetables are crucial to a healthy diet. You need to feed your body natural food—that is food as nature designed it—if you want your nervous system to function properly.

Here's why:

1. Foods have a higher nutritional value when they are raw. While the pancreas produces many of its own enzymes, you should be consuming enzymes from your food as well. However, temperatures above 112°F can destroy the enzymes that are crucial to thousands of chemical reactions throughout your body. Ironically, many of the enzymes that are destroyed in the heat actually help aid digestion and mineral absorption.

2. The body is normally slightly alkaline at a pH of 7.35-7.45, but cooked foods along with stress, pollutants, and processed, refined goods can raise your acidity level. Unfortunately, higher acidity levels can impair your body's immune system and contribute to the development of respiratory, digestive, and circulatory conditions. Raw foods help to neutralize the acidity in your body and strengthen it against harmful bacteria and viruses.

3. Raw foods are easy to break down, and they don't linger on their way through the digestive system. Foods that are difficult to process often ferment causing toxins to accumulate in the gut. When foods ferment, the fats go rancid, the proteins putrefy, and the mucosal linings of the intestines become inflamed. On a raw food diet, you'll be less likely to suffer from digestive disorders like gas, heartburn, constipation and indigestion.

4. A raw food diet is great for your overall health and has even been shown to have a positive effect on chronic diseases like cancer, heart disease, and, in my case, tinnitus.

    Antioxidants prevent damage done by floating free radicals, or single oxygen molecules. Your body needs free radicals to fight off viruses and microbes, but a surplus can cause the body a great deal of harm.

    Fruits and vegetables high in antioxidants happen to be particularly sensitive to heat because the phytonutrients found in them can't survive high temperatures. Phytonutrients normally protect plants from dangerous environments, but they can be damaged by radiation, pollution, and pesticides. Moreover, as it turns out, we as humans need phytonutrients for many of the same reasons plants do!

5. A diet rich in raw foods gives you the vitamins your body needs to protect itself from common illnesses like colds and flus. Even common viruses deplete the body of energy and resources it could surely use for more productive purposes. Raw food helps to keep the systems of the body functioning the way they were meant to.

    You by no means have to forego your cooked dishes to benefit from raw food either. A couple pieces of fruit and a fresh salad for lunch can still boost your body's immune system and provide it with the nutrients it needs to fight off tinnitus. The phrase "raw food" doesn't have to imply a trendy fad diet just because some have decided to adopt the diet in its extreme form.

    Whether you decide to start adding more fresh produce to your daily routine or you take a few weeks to go on a raw food cleanse, you should definitely consider incorporating more raw food into your diet if you're serious about overcoming tinnitus.

What You Should Eat

A raw food diet is not necessarily made up solely of raw foods. The goal of the diet is to eat the foods in as close to their whole state as possible. That means either eating them as they are or simply boiling or steaming them until they're soft enough to eat. In any case, you'll want to avoid foods that are highly processed. So, if you want to eat rice, for example, go with brown rice as opposed to white rice.

Here's just a partial list of foods that we consider raw: whole grain cereals, legumes, fermented soy products, fruits, vegetables, sea vegetables – like seaweed, brown rice, soba noodles, all types of beans, and tofu. You may have noticed a lack of meat; this is deliberate. By and large, a raw diet does not include meat; only raw fish and other seafood are allowed. That being said, you'll want to avoid eating peppers, potatoes, tomatoes, spinach, beets, avocadoes, and eggplant in excess.

Even though coffee and soda are permitted, you'll want to avoid drinking too much caffeine. It's best to stick to mostly water if possible.

While you're eating, make sure to keep your portions small and chew your food well. Breaking food up into small, manageable amounts puts less stress on your digestive system.

When preparing your plate, take the following guidelines into account: first, make about half your meal of whole grains, including brown rice. This is especially important if you have an allergy to gluten, as rice is gluten-free. Next, you'll want about a third of the meal to be vegetables. Beans and legumes can make up ten percent and soup five percent. To round things out, toss in some nuts, fish, juices and seasoning as you see fit. You really want to avoid red meat as much as possible. If you really like meat and feel that you need some, at least aim to buy meat that was raised locally. In fact, when it comes to all of your foods, try to get only local produce.

Follow these guidelines, and you're sure to see a real improvement in the state of your overall health.

The Health Benefits of a Raw Food Diet

If the idea of a raw diet conjures up images of half-starved, organic-loving rabbits living somewhere within the vicinity of San Francisco, you might want to reconsider. Many of the healthiest diets in the world are comprised heavily of raw food. Raw fish and seaweed is a staple in the Oriental world, and the Mediterranean diet is full of fresh veggies stuffed into falafel, dipped in hummus, or simply eaten on their own. Step into any hotel in Tel Aviv and you'll find the breakfast buffet lined with fresh salads dressed elegantly with a simple drizzle of olive oil. The western world has conditioned us to believe wholeheartedly in the power of fried chicken, melted cheese, and thick-crust pizza, but the raw food diet is far from rare. Here are some of the health benefits of the raw food diet you may not have considered.

1. *Protect against diseases*

Because they're water soluble, vitamins B and C will often dissolve into a pot of hot water. If you're boiling your vegetables into oblivion, you may be losing some of these essential vitamins. Vitamin C is a powerful antioxidant that destroys free radicals floating around in the body and nitrates, preservatives often contained in packaged foods, both of which are known to lead to cancer. It also supports healthy immune function and combats common colds and viruses.

2. *Weight maintenance*

A raw food diet can help you maintain a healthy body weight because it focuses on low-fat, natural ingredients. Raw fruits and vegetables naturally contain fewer calories even when they're eaten in abundance. More importantly though, they don't contain refined oils and saturated fats you find in butter, lard, and many cooking oils. These fats are known to clog arteries putting you at a higher risk for heart disease and diabetes. Fried foods are particularly unhealthy not only because they're high in calories, because also they're high in trans fats, a compound that's very difficult for the body to break down.

3. *No More Heartburn*

Heartburn is a condition of the esophagus caused by excess stomach acid. Normally the body has a neutral and even a slightly alkaline pH. However, stress, pollutants, refined foods, and mineral-deficient water can drastically affect the pH balance in the body. Raw fruits and vegetables neutralize these acids thereby returning the body to homeostasis and minimizing heartburn and indigestion.

4. *Increased Energy-*

If you've ever passed out on the couch after Thanksgiving dinner, you know how lethargic you feel following a large meal made of biscuits, gravy, turkey, and pumpkin pie. Besides the sheer amount of calories you would have consumed, these foods are likely to make you drowsy simply because they are so heavy and difficult for the body to digest.

Moreover, the average western diet contains far too many grains and pastas, which cause the blood sugar levels to spike and then crash suddenly. Without as many refined carbohydrates, your energy levels will remain more stable throughout the day. By contrast, raw fruits and vegetables are easily digestible and are packed with the vitamins and minerals you need to stay energized and focused for hours on end.

On a second note, the vitamin B complex, which is water soluble as I mentioned above, is responsible for converting food into energy to support normal metabolic function and healthy brain development. If you're deficient in vitamin B, you should notice fatigue and a lack of mental clarity. Since this vitamin is water soluble, your body won't store it; instead, you'll excrete it through urine.

So, you need to consume enough of it on a regular basis to keep your body energized and your mind focused. Interestingly enough though, vitamin B isn't readily available in many leafy greens because they contain oxalates, an acid commonly found in plants that blocks absorption of certain minerals in the gut. Make sure that you lightly steam these veggies to reduce the oxalate count. Just remember to keep the temperature below 112°F to keep it raw.

https://www.tricitymed.org/2018/08/b-vitamins-secret-good-skin-health/
https://www.healthline.com/nutrition/10-proven-benefits-of-kale#bottom-line
https://www.healthline.com/nutrition/oxalate-good-or-bad #TOC_TITLE_HDR_10

The Healthy Way To Do Raw Food Diets

Years ago, nutritionists were touting the benefits of the grapefruit diet as a miracle cure to lose weight quickly and effectively. If you ate nothing but grapefruit, indeed a diet that was cleverly named, you would shed pounds by the day. Of course, in reality you would lose weight because you'd become so fed up with the citrus fruit you'd simply throw down your fork and abandon the fruit altogether.

Alas, grapefruit in excess is not healthy at all. Not only does this diet seriously lack essential nutrients, but it contains an overwhelming amount of acid that will destroy your teeth and upset your pH balance. Don't make the same mistake and assume you can simply eat anything you want in whatever quantity simply because you're eating primarily fruits and vegetables. The raw diet, like any other diet, demands moderation. Here are some guidelines to help you maintain a balanced lifestyle.

Eat Locally

Because of today's incredible economy, you can easily go to the supermarket and find food grown on the other side of the country or even the other side of the world. Locally grown food is of course somewhat limited in variety. However, produce from farms in your area will be fresher and healthier than crops that have been imported.

Usually locally grown goods contain fewer pesticides, but more importantly, they haven't travelled as far to get to your plate. Fruits and vegetables develop many of their nutrients as they're ripening, but in order to ship them to you, farmers will harvest the produce weeks before these crops reach maturity. On top of that, commercial farms will treat the fruits and vegetables with chemicals to prevent them from ripening on their long journey thereby preventing many of the nutrients from forming at all. By the time they arrive at your fridge, they're depleted of many of the nutrients they would have had if they been in transit for only 24-48 hours.

Limit Dried Fruits

Dried fruit contains a large amount of sugar in each serving, and because the food is relatively concentrated, it's easy to consume double or triple your recommended daily intake. While dried fruit is a healthy source of fiber and key vitamins and minerals, sugar is still sugar. Fructose, in excessive doses can wreak havoc on blood sugar levels, send the metabolism into overdrive, and wear away at the enamel on your teeth. While a small handful of raisins is perfectly fine, be careful to measure out portion sizes and not snack on dried fruit absentmindedly.

Don't Go Nuts

Because the raw diet is naturally low in calories, it can be easy to turn to nuts in an attempt to satisfy your hunger. Nuts are a healthy source of protein, fat, and calories, but eaten in excess, they pose a threat to your digestive system. While the fat present in nuts is generally unsaturated, an entire bag of nuts for lunch won't do any favors for your waistline. Moreover, nuts contain dietary fiber that can cause bloating, diarrhea, and gas if abused.

Get the Right Advice

Just because your best friend had great results with her raw food diet doesn't necessarily mean the same advice will apply equally to you. Your body is different and will respond differently to the same food. While her advice may be sincere and well-intentioned, it's imperative that you consult with a doctor or a qualified health professional. He/She will be able to provide suggestions tailored specifically to your needs based on your family history, dietary sensitivities, allergies, current medications, and any other medical conditions that may affect your nutritional requirements.

If you follow these simple guidelines, you'll avoid many of the pitfalls that plague raw dieters.

https://greenopedia.com/local-food-is-healthier/

To Cook or Not to Cook?

Did you know that human beings are the only creatures on Earth that heat up their food before eating it? Think about it: do you know of any animals that whip out their spatula when they start to get a bit hungry? Just because members of the animal kingdom eat a certain way doesn't necessarily mean we should too—after all, we're also the only species that plays chess, regularly does the laundry, and washes dirt off our food before eating it.

That being said, are there benefits to cooking? What do we stand to gain from a raw diet, and, as an extension, are there situations in which cooking food is actually preferable? We've talked about most of the pros and cons already, but we thought we'd clearly lay out all of the reasons on both side of the argument for you.

Why Go Raw?

Why exactly should you go raw? Whether it's for a week or a few months, the raw diet may help you get back on track.

1. *Preserve Water Soluble Vitamins*
    When boiling vegetables, many of the water-soluble vitamins, like vitamins B and C as well as thiamin, riboflavin, niacin, and folate are lost to the pot of water. The amount lost while cooking will vary depending on the temperature, the amount of water, and the cooking time, but leafy greens, for example, can lose up to 40% of their vitamin C.
2. *Higher Nutrient Intake*
    You may very well have no problem fulfilling your daily dietary requirements, but the standard American diet is severely lacking in nutrients. Reverting to a raw diet even for a week or two forces you to rely on foods that are very nutrient dense. If your diet primarily contains fruit, vegetables, and nuts, you're far more likely to get the vitamins and minerals your body may have been lacking otherwise. If your breakfast consists of a green smoothie and your dinner a hearty salad, you'll quickly pack in nutrients that your body needs.
3. *Greater Variety of Fruits and Vegetables*
    We all have our favorites—some of us like broccoli, some of us prefer carrots, but the single serving of vegetables with dinner won't provide much variety. Carrots are good. Broccoli is too. The point though is that you should be eating all different kinds of fruits and vegetables especially if you want to support healthy nervous system function.
4. *Limit Oils, Salts, and Sugars*
    When we cook, we sometimes use oils and salts and even sugars a bit too liberally. While oils and salts are permitted in a raw diet, you're far less likely to lay on the oil if you're not stir frying or roasting your vegetables. Lightly

drizzling a vinaigrette over a fresh salad should be more than enough to coat the leaves. Heavily refined oils have a low oxidation point and are loaded with trans fats. It's easy to abuse even healthy oils like olive oil though, which is very high in fat. Excess salt raises your blood pressure and puts strain on your kidneys while the sugar you might use to season your carrot salad or caramelize red onions is associated with mood swings, anxiety, inflammation, and lower energy levels. These seemingly harmless additives can quickly add up if you're not keeping track even if you're following a vegan diet.

5. *Increased Fiber Intake*

Fiber is absolutely crucial to a healthy digestive system. The recommended daily fiber intake is between 25-38g depending on size and gender. However, according to a study done between 1999-2008 by the Department of Family Medicine in the University of South Carolina, the average American above the age of 18 only consumes between 15g and 18g per day, which, in some cases, is less than half what it should be. You should have absolutely no trouble eating enough fiber on a raw diet, and you might even experience some mild discomfort the first few days as your body learns to cope with added roughage.

6. *Hydrate & Detoxify*

Water is, without a doubt, the most important thing you can put in your body. It helps to flush out wastes, cushion and lubricate joints, facilitate metabolic reactions, regulate the body temperature, and keep mucus passageways moisturized properly. Most importantly, without enough water, your kidneys won't be able to properly filter and flush out toxins as they should. Many of us don't drink as much water as we should, but fresh fruits and vegetables are made up largely of water and can help keep you hydrated even if you've forgotten your water bottle at home.

7. *Take Time to Reset*

Sometimes we have to go to an extreme in order to get ourselves back into balance. A standard American diet full of preservatives, additives, chemicals, and refined oils, which put an enormous strain on the digestive system. Even if you don't plan to keep a raw diet forever, you can see it as a way to give your system the chance to hit the reset button. The corn syrup and sugar in our food is addictive, and sometimes eating in moderation is actually more difficult than avoiding the food altogether. A week of raw food will give you the time to nourish your body properly and overcome some bad eating habits.

Benefits of Cooking

1. *Tomatoes*

Turns out the Italians knew what they were doing when they started making tomato sauce. When cooked, tomatoes release the antioxidant lycopene, which has been associated with lower risks of cancer and heart attack. Lycopene is a carotenoid responsible for the tomato's red color, and since it's an incredibly powerful antioxidant, even if cooking the tomato reduces its Vitamin C levels, the added lycopene will make it worth it.

2. *Carrots*

Studies have shown that carrots have higher levels of beta-carotene than raw carrots. The body converts beta-carotene into vitamin A, which, in turn, aids in vision, immune function, bone growth, and reproduction.

3. *Oxalates*

A beautiful spinach salad with a vibrant vinaigrette from time to time is a treat, but you're missing key nutrients if you only eat raw spinach. Spinach is known to contain relatively large amounts of oxalic acid, an acid that typically found in plants that blocks absorption of certain minerals in the gut. You'll need to heat spinach to reduce the oxalates in the food.

4. *More Palatable*

Some vegetables are simply not palatable raw, but you shouldn't forsake pumpkin, squash, potatoes, and asparagus simply because they're cooked. Cooking helps to break down their cell walls rendering their antioxidants and vitamins more available for absorption.

There are plenty of important reasons for cooking your food, but they certainly don't outweigh the benefits of eating raw. Increasing the amount of raw food in your diet can jumpstart your metabolism, boost your energy levels, and give your body the nutrients it needs to function at peak performance.

Why to Avoid Heat in the Kitchen

When you were a child, your parents probably warned you never to play with matches, and for good reason too. They certainly didn't want you to burn yourself! That's also why your mom and dad would have told you to lather up every time you went out to the beach. Protection from the sun is equally important. Not only are sunburns painful, but exposure to the sun in excessive amounts can put you at risk for skin cancer.

As it turns out, you won't want to burn your food either.

Smoke in the kitchen should be a sign of disaster for any chef, but ironically and perhaps quite unfortunately, charring, broiling, and browning is often the technique of choice. Grill marks decorating a sizzling steak are the ultimate sign of a drool-worthy meal as demonstrated by any number of restaurant commercials. It's not only meat though that people will eat blackened. Browning onions or citrus fruits, for instance, lends the fruit or vegetable a deep, earthy flavor. The produce gives soups and stews a degree of intensity it wouldn't have otherwise. Whether it's scorched marshmallows, a charred chicken cutlet, or burnt sugar across the top of crème brûlée, burnt food is more common than you might have otherwise assumed.

Charred meats smoking over an open grill—is it an integral part of the barbecue experience? Perhaps, but when protein-rich foods are cooked at very high temperatures, they release heterocyclic amines (HCA's), which has been linked to increase risk in breast, colon, liver, skin, lung, and prostate cancer by the National Cancer Institute. Polycyclic aromatic hydrocarbons (PAH's) will form from fat dripping from the grill, and even if it doesn't touch your meat directly, the smoke from the burning oil will ultimately affect the food anyway. PAH-rich diets have been linked to leukemia, GI, and lung cancer. In fact, if you consume well-done meat on a regular basis, you raise your risk of developing pancreatic cancer by a whopping 60% according to a 9-year study of 62,000 people conducted by the University of Minnesota.

You're not necessarily safe with charred vegetables either though. Cooking starchy vegetables and grains at high temperatures produces acrylamide, a chemical associated with cancer in animals. The link hasn't yet been proven with humans, but the Food Standards Agency (FSA) of the U.K. has already issued warnings against consuming burned foods. Whether baked, fried, grilled, toasted, or roasted, blackened fruits and vegetables contain high levels of acrylamide specifically if they have a high sugar content.

Though scientists don't know how much of the chemical the human body can tolerate over an extended period of time, eating a raw diet full of fruits and vegetables is a surefire way to avoid many of the starchy breads, pastas, baked goods, and processed foods that expose you to this potentially fatal compound.

You also won't want to forget about the oil you might be using to cook. Just because oil is a liquid doesn't mean it can't burn. Once an oil reaches its smoking point, it begins to release free-radical, a harmful, reactive substance that is potentially cancerous if left unchecked. It will also release acrolein, the chemical that gives burnt food its acrid taste.

Many of the healthier oils like virgin olive oil happen to have a particularly low smoking points because they're very refined food products full of minerals and enzymes. In fact, you really should reserve these oils for dressing salads or drizzling over a bowl of hummus. Between 325-375°F, virgin olive oil already begins to break down. If you use oil to deep fry food, you have to take precautions to keep the temperature under control. Oil heats up very quickly, and you may not realize how quickly the temperature is rising as the pot sits on the burner.

The black char marks of a perfectly grilled sweet pepper may be attractive, but heat can drastically change the nature of a food sometimes for the worse. While cooking isn't all bad, it very well might be the enemy of food in some cases. If you are cooking, you'll want to stick with the textbook golden brown if you want to make sure to limit the amount of toxins in your bloodstream. Better yet, stick with steaming vegetables at lower temperatures to avoid the many harmful effects of high heat.

https://www.health.com/steam-vs-boil-vegetables-8743881

Finding The Ingredients For Your Raw Food Diet

Despite the numerous benefits associated with the raw food diet, actually transitioning from your current diet can be difficult to say the least. Thankfully, finding the ingredients for your new meals is easier than you may think.

Because Americans are becoming increasingly aware of their health choices, specialty markets and organic food stores like Whole Foods and Trader Joe's seem to be popping up all across the country. If you happen to live in a big city, you're likely to have a larger range of options than you might have even realized. Even if you live in a smaller urban area or out in the suburbs, you shouldn't have any trouble finding at least a couple health boutiques if you're willing to search for them.

If not though, never fear. Your regular grocery store should carry more than enough produce for your raw food needs. During the spring and summer months, you might even be able to find fruits and vegetables grown at local farms. The grocery store should also have a wide selection of dried and frozen fruit, sprouts, bagged nuts, and seeds. It might be slightly more difficult to find raw grains, but you should at least be able to purchase dried oats, which are located in the cereal section. If you can't find raw grains at the supermarket or at specialty stores, you can easily order them online and have them shipped right to your home.

If your grocery store doesn't carry fresh, organic produce or the produce just doesn't happen to be to your liking, you can frequent farmer's markets. Farmers will either sell their crops at a stand at the road side or at the local farmer's market. Check the newspaper to find out more information about farmers markets in your area. Usually they are held at least a couple of times a week at a central location. Not only is the produce far cheaper and fresher, but it's also sold in bulk. Unfortunately, the fruits and vegetables need to be washed carefully before consumption because they often still contain pesticide residue.

Once you start your regular shopping trips, you might notice that your weekly food bill is substantially lower. Even if you regularly indulge in organic produce, you'll still save yourself a hefty chunk of change every year if you're not buying animal products.

Cheaper still, grow your own garden. With a shovel and a green thumb you can grow all of the ingredients you need right in your own backyard. Besides, growing your own garden is the only sure-fire way to monitor exactly what pesticides and chemicals go into your food. Tomatoes, zucchini, green beans, carrots, and strawberries are particularly easy plants to start with, and the potted plants look lovely on a back patio. Better yet, toiling the land is gratifying, rewarding experience. You'll never appreciate your food more than when you grow it yourself.

General Raw Food Dietary Guidelines

The Raw Vegan diet contains three essential food groups, and understanding these three food groups is your key to healthy meal-planning. You should regularly be partaking of leafy green vegetables, sweet fruits, and high-fat plants in relatively balanced amounts.

There is a range of opinions regarding what percentage of your diet should come from leafy green vegetables. I've read that these greens should make up as little as 2% and as much as 30% of your diet. It's highly unlikely that you can eat between 500-700 calories in green vegetables unless you plan on eating salad all day long. Fortunately, you can derive the benefits of leafy green vegetables from a relatively modest amount.

500 grams per day should be more than enough to get plenty of calcium, protein, vitamin K, and zinc. While 500g is still a lot, you can always mix your greens into smoothies or grind them into pesto if you find you're having a hard time meeting your daily requirement. Despite popular belief, vegetables and leafy greens in particular are loaded with calcium that can strengthen your bones and teeth and can even help lower blood pressure.

There's no specified amount of fruit you should eat per day, but you should exercise discretion. Fruit eaten in excess will wear down the teeth because it contains large amounts of sugar and acid. When choosing your fruit, feel free to eat whatever is in season. There's no need to turn to expensive or exotic fruits—the fresh fruit at your local supermarket should suffice. For instance, bananas are high in potassium, and oranges provide plenty of calcium, folate, potassium, and vitamin C.

Without enough high-fat plant foods, you won't ingest the calories you need to maintain your weight. Vegetable oils, olives, avocados, nuts, and potatoes are all healthy sources of monounsaturated fat that will provide you with the energy your body requires on a daily basis. Up to 40% of your diet should come from high-fat plant foods if you intend to meet your regular caloric requirements.

High-fat plant foods are an excellent source of omega-3, an essential fatty acid that regulates eye and brain health, reduces inflammation, and can even mitigate the effects of depression. You can find omega-3 fatty acids in flax seeds. Simply drizzle a bit of flax seed oil over your salad dressing for a power-packed lunch.

Lastly, you'll have to find ways to include enough B12 in your diet. B12 is found overwhelmingly in meat, fish, and eggs, and vegans often find it difficult to consume enough on a regular basis. There are natural sources of B12 in wild plants such as nori and spirulina, but if those aren't available, you might have to rely on a supplement.

Health experts generally only recommend supplements or pills as a last resort if you really cannot get enough B12 from your regular diet. You can always turn to probiotics and fermented foods though. However, make sure to consult with your doctor immediately if you start noticing headaches, weakness, dizziness, breathlessness, mood changes, and disturbed vision. Untreated, a serious vitamin B12 deficiency can result in anemia and damage to the nervous system.

With these guidelines, you can plan healthy, balanced meals that will keep you feeling at your best and hopefully minimize the effects of tinnitus quickly and efficiently.

Raw Plant Protein vs. Animal Protein

Usually when the word protein comes up, the word "meat" springs to mind almost immediately afterward. We've been brought up to believe that chicken, beef, and pork are the ideal sources of protein especially if eaten in large quantities. Moreover, the dairy industry has done a wonderful job of convincing us that a healthy, balanced diet contains three servings of dairy a day. While this information isn't necessarily false, it can be misleading because proteins derived from plant sources are just as valuable, if not more so, than animal-derived ones.

Though there are some notable exceptions, plant foods, for the most part, do not contain all 20 amino acids, and that's why we refer to them as incomplete. It's important that you consume all amino acids because your body cannot produce them on its own. However, even though you can't find all 20 amino acids in very many foods, you should still eat your fill if you consume a variety of plant foods. That is to say that individual vegetables contain fewer amino acids, but you can still find the entire spectrum of amino acids within the plant kingdom.

On the other hand, animal proteins, when eaten in excess, can be very dangerous for a number of reasons. First of all, eating proteins with a higher proportion of amino acids causes the body to release the hormone insulin-like growth factor-1 (IGF-1) in higher quantities. Because this hormone causes cells to reproduce, its often linked with the cancer.

That's not the only growth hormone released because of animal proteins though. Animal protein also contains higher levels of phosphorus. To counterbalance the higher levels of phosphorus, the body produces a different growth hormone: fibroblast growth factor-23 (FGF23). FGF23 is oftentimes linked with hypertrophy of the cardiac ventricle, a condition that leads to heart attack, heart failure, and sudden death.

Animal proteins are also associated with higher levels of trimethylamine N-oxide (TMAO), a substance created in the gut that damages the inner linings of organs and tissues and aids in the growth of cholesterol plaques in the blood vessels. They also contain higher sulfur-containing amino acids, which, when metabolized, cause the digestive system to become more acidic. When the pH in our bodies is too low, our bodies often draw calcium from the bones to neutralize the acid unfortunately weakening our bones in the process.

Last but not least, animal foods contain higher levels of heme-iron, as opposed to plant foods, which contain non-heme iron. Heme-iron is known to convert oxidants into highly reactive free-radicals, which damage protein structures and ultimately lead to cancer when not eliminated by antioxidants. Heme-iron absorbs more quickly than non-heme iron, but because the body only needs iron in limited quantities, iron from a plant-based diet should be more than sufficient.

This all goes without saying that animal proteins also contain higher cholesterol and lower fiber. The body produces more than enough HDL cholesterol on its own, and LDL cholesterol and saturated fat congeals in the blood vessels, one of the most common causes of heart disease in the United States. Fiber helps combat colon and breast cancer and may even reduce stroke and heart attack. Yet most adults eat less than half of their daily recommended amount of the nutrient that helps to neutralize the effects of high cholesterol. The irony would be humorous if the consequences weren't so grave.

Ultimately, it's easy for carnivores to pick at protein levels as the most obvious argument against vegetarianism and veganism. According to the American Dietetic Association though, people only need about 0.8g per kilogram of bodyweight. Unless you're a serious athlete, you shouldn't have to worry excessively about consuming enough protein. However, overconsumption of protein can lead to digestive issues, mineral imbalances, and even growth of cancer. It's unfortunately true that many plant eaters don't take the time to plan balanced meals, but a diligent vegan should have no trouble consuming the proper amount of protein. It's animal-eaters we should really be worrying about.

https://www.forksoverknives.com/animalproteindangers/#gs.r_sXUtg
https://www.health.harvard.edu/blog/how-much-protein-do-you-need-every-day-201506188096
https://www.healthline.com/nutrition/animal-vs-plant-protein

How to Cook When You Need To

There's something simply more appealing about raw experiences. Whether it's raw power, raw sex, or even a raw wound, the word exposes the intensity inherent in life's most pivotal moments. We, as humans, like what is natural, unrefined, and unaffected, and the same goes for the food we eat. Our bodies crave the fruit of the earth—the gifts mother nature created specifically to fuel our bodies.

The nutrients in raw food cannot be manufactured, preserved, or artificially created in the boxes, cans, or bottles that sit in our pantries for weeks on end. The idea of canned fish or microwavable meals shouldn't sound appetizing to anyone. Nonetheless, we tend to live our lives out of the can these days. It's only too easy on busy evenings to turn to frozen pizza and canned peas because it's far easier than cooking dinner properly. Just because today we can quickly fill our grumbling stomachs though doesn't mean our bodies are getting the nutrients they need.

Your body, and perhaps even more importantly your brain, needs the vitamins that are found in raw produce.

That being said, it's not always easy to eat all vegetables raw. Asparagus, for instance, needs to be cooked before it can be consumed because it contains too much roughage for our bodies to digest easily. Thankfully though, there are ways to cook vegetables while minimizing the damage caused by heat.

As a general rule, you'll want to keep cooking times to a minimum. The ideal way to cook your vegetables is to steam them because you can keep both the cooking time and the temperature to a minimum. When you boil vegetables, the water tends to drain the vitamin B, vitamin C, and folate from the food into the water. So, unless you plan on drinking the water as well, like you would if you were making soup or stew, you'll want to opt for steaming over boiling.

As a last resort, you can also roast or grill your vegetables. While you do have to cook the vegetables at a high temperature, you won't be losing any water-soluble vitamins in the process. Just make sure to keep the temperature below the smoking point of the oil you use and go easy on the salt. Refined oils, such as extra virgin olive oil, burn at 410°F, and salt lowers the boiling point even further. When heated to its smoking point, oil will release harmful free-radicals and change in flavor.

So, eat your raw veggies, but remember that a little heat here and there can actually be beneficial if used in moderation. Besides, not all of your nutrients need to come from raw food anyway. 80% of your caloric intake is more than enough, and better yet, if you vary your cooking methods, you won't lose too much of any one nutrient anyway

Fruits & Vegetables With the Highest Pesticide Levels

We all know that farmers spray their foods with pesticides to ward off pesky insects and other irritating pests, but few of us know to what degree. While the Department of Agriculture reports that the pesticide residue left on our food poses no risk to our health, the public thinks otherwise. According to Consumer Reports, over 85%

of the 1,000 people surveyed were concerned about the chemicals left on their fruits and vegetables.

In fact, the Organic Trade Association claims that 51% of families are choosing more organic produce than they were in 2014. So, are these numbers just a fluke, or is there real reason to believe the hype? Between 2005 and 2014, sales for organic produce rose from $5.4 billion to a stunning $35.9 billion, a clear and obvious sign that Americans don't trust commercial farms like they used to.

As it turns out, yes. While the Department of Agriculture reports human tolerance levels for individual pesticides, the majority of fruit you find in your supermarket contains more than one. However, there is currently no medical research on the synergistic effects of pesticides.

A survey sent out by the Food Safety and Sustainability Center claims that up to 1/3 of Americans believe that the laws set out by the government safely regulate the chemicals that are found on their food. However, in reality, almost 1/3 of fruits and vegetables that undergo the USDA's testing are found to contain residue from at least two different kinds of pesticide if not more. **The effects of these combinations are unknown and untested.**

Because organic produce is quite pricey though, you'll need to know which food typically contain the highest levels of pesticides. Thankfully, the Environmental Working Group (EWG) tests produce every year and releases what they call the Dirty Dozen list. These twelve fruits and vegetables contain the highest levels of pesticides even once they reach the shelves of your local grocery store. These results from the 2015 survey can help you to make the right decisions to keep your family happy and healthy.

1. *Apples*

That's right, the red empire's you send in your child's lunchbox are #1 on the list. In fact, 99% of apples that they tested came back with chemical residue. When the FDA tested grocery store apples in 2012, they found a stunning 36 different chemicals, and at least 18 of these chemicals are neurotoxins known to cause brain damage.

2. *Peaches*

The EWG reported that 98% of peaches tested positive for at least one pesticide, and unfortunately, the skin offers little to no protection from these harmful chemicals. Farmers regularly apply up to 45 different kinds of pesticides to their peach crops, so chances are fairly high you'll encounter more than one when picking up these fuzzy fruits.

3. *Nectarines*

Out of all the nectarines tested, 97% of them contained residue for at least one toxin.

4. *Strawberries*

U. S. farmers pour 300 pounds of pesticides to each acre of their strawberry crops. That means that each individual berry contains 36 different kinds of chemicals. Just think of that when you're making your strawberry jam this summer. V.

5. *Grapes*

A single grape may contain up to 15 different pesticides, but you'll find a total of 35 different chemicals used throughout the surrounding vineyards.

6. *Celery*

Celery contains no peel, and so the 29 different chemicals used to keep away bugs soak right into the stem itself.

7. *Spinach*

Just because your spinach says triple-washed doesn't necessarily mean your safe. This salad favorite was loaded with toxins in 88% of the samples taken.

8. *Sweet Bell Peppers*

A single basket of sweet bell peppers can contain up to 15 different pesticides, but up to 88 different pesticides were found in all.

9. *Cucumbers*

One cucumber contained up to 10 different pesticides.

10. *Cherry Tomatoes*

According to the FDA, farmers employ more than 30 different pesticides on their tomatoes, but the skin does nothing to prevent these toxins from penetrating the fruit. On a single fruit, you might find up to 13 chemicals.

11. *Snap Peas*

Snap peas also tested positive for 13 different pesticides.

12. *Potatoes*

Only 91% of potatoes were found to contain one or more pesticides, but by weight, this root vegetable actually contains more pesticides than all of the other foods on the list.

Lastly, raspberries were found to contain 39 chemicals with 58% of them testing positive for pesticides, while a single cherry contained up to 25 toxins.

Fortunately, there are *some* clean foods. The 2015 report found that only 1% of avocados were contaminated. 61% of cantaloupes and 80% of papayas, pineapples, kiwi, and mangos were totally chemical free. Finally, cabbage, frozen sweet peas, asparagus, grapefruit, sweet potatoes, sweet corn, onions, eggplant, and cauliflower were also relatively safe.

If you indulge on anything this year, you'll want to indulge on organic produce. The extra few dollars you spend every week will keep your children's bodies and minds healthy and safe. Indeed, with thousands of chemicals used on your fresh produce every year, you can't afford to take any risks.

How Poor Diet Choices Affect Hormone Balance

Hormones are the chemical messengers that regulate nearly all metabolic functions including immune response, menstruation and sperm production, blood sugar levels, and moods and emotional reactions.

We typically refer to hormone imbalances with regards to the female reproductive system because women are accustomed to experiencing hormone fluctuation. Whether during menstruation, pregnancy, breastfeeding, or menopause, a woman's hormones will shift dramatically throughout her life. Though hormones are crucial to sexual health for both men and women, their work extends to all areas of human health.

The food and household objects you have lying around your kitchen can have enormous impact on your endocrine system. In this sense, whether you're struggling with tinnitus or you're simply trying to improve your health, you'll need to be more vigilant about what you allow into your home and into your body.

Phthalates

You're probably consuming phthalates every single day without even knowing it. This class of chemical compounds is used to make plastics soft and pliable—think of the rubber ducky you have in your bathtub. Because they hold onto scent and color well, they're commonly used in children's toys, perfumes, cosmetics, and plastic food and drink containers.

Phthalates are practically everywhere. Not only are they in the food we eat and the soap we wash with, but they're even in the air. If you're not absorbing them through your skin, you're inhaling them when you breathe.

While moderate phthalate levels in the blood stream are to be expected, higher levels are associated with birth defects, lower sperm counts, thyroid problems, diabetes, and obesity.

To limit your exposure to these chemicals, you'll want to avoid storing your food in plastic containers, skip the plastic water bottles, and limit the number of plastic chew toys you give to your young children. Watch out for cosmetics with "fragrance" in the ingredients list; in fact, limiting the amount of personal care products you use in general can greatly lower your phthalate levels.

BPA

BPA is an industrial chemical used to make polycarbonate plastics stronger. However, because not all of it is sealed in properly, it typically leaks from metal cans into the foods you consume. It's found in canned foods, toiletries, feminine hygiene products, and household electronics.

BPA mimics the sex hormones the body produces naturally, and so it binds to receptors designed for estrogen, testosterone, etc. These endocrine disruptors are very dangerous because they hinder crucial metabolic reactions. High levels of BPA can be traced to early onset of puberty in adolescents, breast cancer, heart disease, obesity, and cancer of the reproductive organs.

Any food goods or plastics made with BPA will likely be marked with a "PC" (polycarbonate). Alternatively, the recycling sign on products made with BPA will be labeled with either a 3 or a 7. Unfortunately, more than 90% of people have a detectable amount of this chemical in their bloodstream. However, you can lower the level of BPA in your body dramatically simply by limiting your use of pre-packaged or canned goods.

Dioxin

Dioxin is an organic chemical related to DDT produced by the burning of PVC plastics, creation of bleached paper, and the use of certain herbicides. It does not degrade in the environment, and it accumulates in the fat cells of animals over time preventing them from reproducing.

While the degree of toxicity is not certain, Dioxin can disrupt the endocrine systems and give rise to cancer and immune dysfunction. Dioxin can also be passed to an unborn fetus through the uterus or a newborn through breastmilk. A baby boy introduced to high levels of dioxin will show lower a sperm count and poorer sperm quality.

These toxins are also frequently found in animal products. Dioxin-contaminated meat and dairy products can expose humans to the chemical in large doses. Eating organic produce and switching to a mostly vegetarian diet can help you limit your exposure to these toxins.

Perchlorate

Typically found in rocket fuel, batteries, explosives, fireworks, fertilizers, and airbags, this chemical, which the EPA has   long since labelled as toxic, may also be found in your milk and cheese.

Perchlorate resembles halogens like chlorine, fluorine, and bromine, which are all harmful. Like the other halogens, perchlorate competes with iodine in the thyroid. Thyroid receptors will recognize halogens as iodine, and the resulting hormone imbalance affects normal thyroid function, which largely regulates the metabolism.

Perchlorate has also been shown to affect brain and organ development in toddlers, infants, and unborn children.

A proper reverse osmosis water filter can help you minimize levels of perchlorate in your home water supply. However, the best way to combat this toxin is to monitor your intake of iodine. Iodized salt can help you maintain normal levels of dietary iodine

Atrazine

Approved for use in the U.S. as far back as 1958, atrazine has since become the second most widely used herbicide in the country.

The over 73 million pounds sprayed on golf courses, food crops, and lawns are responsible for delayed puberty in adolescents, development of breast tumors, prostate cancer, birth defects, impaired sexual development, and infertility. Atrazine is also the reason for abnormal feminization in male marine animals. In fact, 85% of American male smallmouth bass are carrying eggs today

The same chemical that is wreaking havoc on the environment is quickly leaking into our water supply and cornfields. The only way to avoid this toxin is to drink filtered water and avoid non-organic corn products.

Lead

Lead is a toxic metal found in the Earth's crust. The widespread use of lead has negatively influenced the environment and put too many people at risk particularly pregnant women and young children.

Because it affects sex hormones, lead is known to cause miscarriages, premature births, still-births, and birth defects. Children can suffer profound, long-term brain and nervous damage when exposed to lead, but even adults can expect high blood pressure and kidney damage.

Found in old chipped paint, jewelry, stained glass, and any water delivered through pipes joined with lead solder, lead is an ever-present danger. If you want to avoid this dangerous chemical, make sure you have a good water filter and that you change it regularly.

Fire Retardants

The chemicals used on your couch cushions to prevent them from bursting into flames are toxins that have been linked to suppressed thyroid function, reproductive disorders, cancer, immune malfunction, and abnormal brain development in children and unborn babies by way of contaminated breast milk.

Fire retardants are nearly impossible to avoid entirely, and even though many versions have been banned by the U.S. government, you'll still find them in your upholstery. However, you can limit your exposure by dusting regularly and staying out of the house when replacing carpets.

Arsenic

If you eat the seeds of an apple core, you won't start growing an apple tree in your stomach. However, you will have consumed a miniscule amount of arsenic. Arsenic is found in many foods and is commonly found in drinking water, but it's not lethal in such low concentrations.

That being said, if enough accumulates, arsenic can lead to various types of cancer, such as bladder, lung, and skin cancer. It also interferes with your body's glucocorticoids so that you can expect weight changes, immune malfunction, protein wastage, insulin resistance, childhood growth retardation, osteoporosis, and high blood pressure.

Make sure to filter your water to eliminate any excess arsenic.

Mercury

Mercury is a toxic metal that has found its way into our environment as a result of pollution and coal-burning industrial power plants.

Mercury mimics some female hormones thereby disturbing menstrual cycles and interfering with normal ovulation. In both sexes, mercury is linked to the development of diabetes because it binds to the islet cells in the pancreas therefore blocking regular insulin function.

Marine life has been heavily affected by high mercury levels, and you should take care to avoid predatory fish like tilefish, king mackerel, shark, swordfish, marlin, orange roughy, ahi tuna, and big-eye tuna. Pregnant women should take extra care to avoid mercury because it can lead to poor brain development in developing fetuses.

PFCs (Per fluorinated Chemicals)

Used to make non-stick cooking equipment, PFC is so prevalent in the environment that virtually everyone has ingested it at one point or another. Some PFCs do not decay naturally in the environment, and so they slowly accumulate over time in our food and water.

PFCs have been linked to low sperm quality, kidney damage, low birth weight, thyroid disease, and high cholesterol. It also interferes with sex hormone levels in both men and women. Unfortunately, the only way to reduce your exposure to PFCs is to avoid non-stick pans and the water-resistant coating often put on furniture, carpets and some clothing.

Organophosphate Pesticides

These pesticides are commonly used on crops to kill pests, and they regularly interfere with testosterone and thyroid hormones.

The best way to avoid organophosphate pesticides is to opt for organic foods as often as possible and to wash fruits and vegetables thoroughly before consuming them.

Glycol Ethers

Glycol ethers are found in cosmetics, brake fluid, cleaning products and paint solvents. They're known to damage the developing reproductive organs of babies while still in uterus through the mother's bloodstream.

Ethyl glycols can also affect the blood and the sperm count in males, and men who are regularly exposed to glycol ethers have been found to have a shrinkage in their testicles. Kids exposed to glycol ethers have an increased risk of allergies and asthma. Plus, it's often found in the paint used to decorate their bedrooms.

Food Additives 101

A food additive is simply anything added to a food during production, processing, or packaging. These predominantly unnatural ingredients are used to increase shelf-life, improve texture, and artificially sweeten diet foods. However, they have nasty side effects that you may not even be aware of.

Additives have been shown to put extra strain on your heart, disrupt your hormone balance, and cause mood shifts and irritability. While the FDA has acted to limit the use of substances it deems harmful, it hasn't acted quickly enough. However, many of these chemicals will linger in your system, slowly accumulating for years. You cannot rely on government agencies to rid the food you eat of these toxins, so unless you're willing to make the effort yourself, you may pay the price later on. Below we've listed the different kinds of preservatives you'll need to watch out for.

Preservatives

Without preservatives, food will spoil in a few days even if it's kept in the refrigerator. Normally, apples turn brown, bread goes moldy, and dairy will grow bacteria. However, these chemicals prevent food from going bad and extend a food's shelf-life far beyond what it would have been otherwise.

Food spoils one of two ways. Sometimes microbes invade and feed off of food's nutrients. If you eat these bacteria, you could develop serious diseases. Otherwise, a chemical change occurs in the food's molecules known as oxidation in which enzymes and free radicals turn fats rancid. Oxidation causes produce like apples and potatoes to turn brown.

Preservatives make it impossible for microbes to survive and thrive off of the food's nutrients. Acids are often used because they destroy the enzymes microbes need to survive. The sorbic acid used in cheese, benzoic acid used in salad dressing, and propionic acid used in baked goods help to do just that.

Antioxidants like BHT and tocopherol prevent chemical changes from taking place. These chemicals are used to sop up the free radicals that cause food to go bad. Another example is ascorbic acid, which is a substitute for vitamin C that staves off browning and helps fruit keep to its color.

Texturizers

Stabilizers, thickeners, and binders are usually added to food to make them more presentable. Emulsifiers, for instance, help blend fatty and watery ingredients smoothly thereby dramatically improving the texture of foods like ice cream.

Other foods you might find in your packaged goods include xanthan gum, guar gum, and carrageenan, which are used as stabilizers and thickeners for low-fat and gluten-free foods.

Acidity Control Additives

Milk, citrus fruits, apples, and plenty of other foods are naturally acidic. However, companies will often add acidity control additives to change or maintain the pH of a product either to prevent the growth of bacteria or add a certain flavor.

Typically indicated by their E number, acidity regulators add flavor to bread, fruit drinks, poultry, pie fillings, wine, jams, and jelly. They may also be used as a thickening agent in cake mixtures and puddings.

Flavoring and Coloring Additives

The food with which mother nature provided us comes in all sorts of vibrant colors and flavors. From bright green to scarlet red, there's hardly a shade you can't find. You can choose from a wide selection of herbs and spices to flavor your food. There's no need to turn to artificial extracts derived from chemicals.

Artificial coloring and dyes are used to create the bright colors you find in sports drinks, candies, and juices. The most common ones you'll see are Red 40, Yellow 5, and Blue 1, and while you might like the bright colors, they're linked to hyperactivity in children.

Choosing Organic

If searching through ingredient lists sounds like too much work, you can always choose organic. Organic foods produced in the U.S. must be free of artificial sweeteners, flavorings, coloring, preservatives, and MSG. Organic crops are grown with natural fertilizers, and farm animals are raised without hormones or antibiotics. So not only are they better for you, but they usually taste better as well.

Final Thoughts:

While many food additives are perfectly safe and sometimes even beneficial, that's generally not the case. You can't go wrong with fresh fruits and vegetables. Remember, if it doesn't decay while sitting on your shelf, it won't when it's in your stomach either. Many food additives aren't degradable, and they remain in your system system for weeks, months, or even years. When in doubt, you can hold by the following maxim: if you cannot pronounce the name, it shouldn't go into your body.

How Organic Eating And Farming Benefits Our Environment

One hundred years ago, no one had ever heard of organic food because these standards were simply the norm. As we've developed the technology to grow food commercially, we've made it easier to produce larger quantities of food, but as a result, we've sacrificed our own health and that of our environment.

How It Helps The Environment

Nature has been in business a long time and it has never needed any of our help. Unfortunately, our society has resorted to manipulating farmland to make it more efficient. However, these commercial farms have depleted our soil of nutrients, contaminated our water supply, started to destroy biodiversity in their areas, and contributed to carbon emissions significantly. Thankfully, organic farming offers us a solution.

1. **Slash Pollution-** The pesticides and chemical fertilizers from commercial farms enters into our water supply as run-off. According to the Organic Trade Association, we could eliminate 500 million pounds of toxins that would otherwise be poured into the environment if every American farmer would just adopt the organic practices.

2. **Preserve Biodiversity-** Because they cannot rely on pesticides to protect their crops organic farmers have to rely on alternative methods of pest control. They're far more likely to encourage birds of prey and other natural predators to keep away insects and rodents. Since organic farmers rely on the environment itself to self-regulate, these farms help to maintain the biodiversity in the area.

3. **Stem the Growth of Super Bacteria-** The widespread use of pesticides and antibiotics promotes the growth of what are commonly referred to as super bacteria. These resistant microbes are not responsive to regular medications and may soon be responsible for the spread of dangerous diseases. If we continue to treat our plants and animals with these chemicals, we are supporting the growth of fungi and bacteria that may end up spreading fatal diseases to humans sometime in the not-so-distant future.

4. **Supports Sustainable Farming-** Organic farming requires the use of healthy, sustainable practices like crop rotation and cover crops. These techniques have been used for centuries to manage erosion and boost soil fertility. Synthetic fertilizers enable plants to grow even when natural conditions would dictate otherwise. As a result, commercial farming helps to deplete the soil of the nutrients and helpful bacteria that should make for healthy crops. Minerals like calcium, potassium, and magnesium that we need to live originally comes from the soil, or at least are supposed to.

5. **Reduce Carbon Emissions-** Without preservatives, organic food won't stay fresh long enough for companies to ship it across the country. So not only will eating organic help to support local agriculture, but it will also reduce carbon emissions that would have resulted from transporting said goods. According to the Rodale Institute Farming Systems Trial of 1981, if only 10,000 American farms adopted organic farming practices, the carbon emissions avoided would be equivalent to removing 1,174,400 cars from the road.

Choose Organic!

By choosing to eat organic food, not only are you nourishing your own body properly, but you might also be helping to preserve the Earth. In a world dominated by pollution, mass production, and commercialization, your choices still matter. After all, this world is our home. If we destroy the environment here, we aren't getting another one. It's our responsibility to take care of our home by making these simple, yet powerful lifestyle choices.

What Does Organic Mean Anyway?

What Does Organic Mean?

Those who have chosen to eat an organic diet know the many positive changes associated with this lifestyle. This seemingly hippy, new age trend is far more realistic and down-to-earth than you might have otherwise imagined.

Organic eating encourages you treat your body and the world around you with the respect it deserves. With a few simple changes and new resolutions, you too can become a more thoughtful and responsible consumer.

What does this mean exactly?

Organic food is defined as food grown in soil free of pesticides, herbicides, hormones, synthetic fertilizers, antibiotics, and other unnatural substances for at least three years prior to planting. Genetic modification is strictly forbidden by the USDA, and in order to receive the USDA stamp of approval, meat must be raised solely on natural pastures and 100% organic feed and forage. No hormones or antibiotics are allowed.

Processed organic foods must be free of artificial preservatives, colors, and flavors and must be made with agricultural ingredients with the exception of pectin in jam, enzymes in yogurt, and baking soda in baked goods.

The organic lifestyle doesn't stop at the kitchen though. Body washes, soaps, creams, lotions, makeup, and shampoos are all manufactured using chemicals and additives that absorb into your skin.

Instead, you'll want to purchase organic personal care products made with essential oils and natural oils such as olive, coconut, lavender, and jojoba. Not only are these items free of chemicals, but they're also usually more effective because they make use of ingredients created by mother nature specifically for our benefit.

Unfortunately, there are no official organic standards for personal care items the way there are in the food industry. Some companies hold by the same standards set by the USDA. Others hold by the National Organic Program (NOP), which lacks the authority to officially regulate organic products. Still others choose to hold by independent standards verified by third parties. Your best bet when shopping for personal care items is to educate yourself about the current rules and regulations.

Lastly, you'll want to purchase or make your own organic cleaning products! Some of the biggest culprits of harsh chemicals and toxins are cleaning products. Your toilet and tub cleaners are usually teaming with harsh chemicals that can be harmful to your skin and possibly to your health.

Ever felt dizzy or nauseous after exposure to cleaning products? Thankfully, there's an easy solution. The best natural cleaners are salt, vinegar, baking soda, and borax, and they can used on just about every inch of your home from the bathroom to the kitchen and on every stain in between.

Organic eating is quickly becoming the new norm in today's society with the organic market bringing in over $35 billion dollars in 2014 in the US alone, which is an 11% increase since 2013. In fact, the organic market has grown by double-digits every year since the 1990s.

51% of families bought more organic products this year than they did in 2014 and 8 in 10 parents choose organic food for their kids. Plus, there are more than 19,500 certified organic farms and processing facilities in the United States alone!

In a world where preservatives, pollution, and industrialization have become the norm, we have an obligation to express our concerns and support clean eating.

What Does Organic Mean Anyway?

What Does Organic Mean?

Those who have chosen to eat an organic diet know the many positive changes associated with this lifestyle. This seemingly hippy, new age trend is far more realistic and down-to-earth than you might have otherwise imagined.

Organic eating encourages you treat your body and the world around you with the respect it deserves. With a few simple changes and new resolutions, you too can become a more thoughtful and responsible consumer.

What does this mean exactly?

Organic food is defined as food grown in soil free of pesticides, herbicides, hormones, synthetic fertilizers, antibiotics, and other unnatural substances for at least three years prior to planting. Genetic modification is strictly forbidden by the USDA, and in order to receive the USDA stamp of approval, meat must be raised solely on natural pastures and 100% organic feed and forage. No hormones or antibiotics are allowed.

Processed organic foods must be free of artificial preservatives, colors, and flavors and must be made with agricultural ingredients with the exception of pectin in jam, enzymes in yogurt, and baking soda in baked goods.

The organic lifestyle doesn't stop at the kitchen though. Body washes, soaps, creams, lotions, makeup, and shampoos are all manufactured using chemicals and additives that absorb into your skin.

Instead, you'll want to purchase organic personal care products made with essential oils and natural oils such as olive, coconut, lavender, and jojoba. Not only are these items free of chemicals, but they're also usually more effective because they make use of ingredients created by mother nature specifically for our benefit.

Unfortunately, there are no official organic standards for personal care items the way there are in the food industry. Some companies hold by the same standards set by the USDA. Others hold by the National Organic Program (NOP), which lacks the authority to officially regulate organic products. Still others choose to hold by independent standards verified by third parties. Your best bet when shopping for personal care items is to educate yourself about the current rules and regulations.

Lastly, you'll want to purchase or make your own organic cleaning products! Some of the biggest culprits of harsh chemicals and toxins are cleaning products. Your toilet and tub cleaners are usually teaming with harsh chemicals that can be harmful to your skin and possibly to your health.

Ever felt dizzy or nauseous after exposure to cleaning products? Thankfully, there's an easy solution. The best natural cleaners are salt, vinegar, baking soda, and borax, and they can used on just about every inch of your home from the bathroom to the kitchen and on every stain in between.

Organic eating is quickly becoming the new norm in today's society with the organic market bringing in over $35 billion dollars in 2014 in the US alone, which is an 11% increase since 2013. In fact, the organic market has grown by double-digits every year since the 1990s.

51% of families bought more organic products this year than they did in 2014 and 8 in 10 parents choose organic food for their kids. Plus, there are more than 19,500 certified organic farms and processing facilities in the United States alone!

In a world where preservatives, pollution, and industrialization have become the norm, we have an obligation to express our concerns and support clean eating.

Complete Guide to Leafy Greens

Known for his great wisdom, Thumper, the loveable hero from *Bambi*, once said, "Greens are a special treat. It makes long ears and great big feet." Truer word were never spoken. Fortunately, if you're not a talking rabbit from an animated Disney film, your feet and ears should remain a normal size despite your intake of these delicious vegetables. Jokes aside, no diet is truly complete without a healthy serving of leafy greens. Not only are they low in calories, but they are loaded with fiber and essential vitamins and minerals.

Whether you layer them onto sandwiches, bake them into casseroles, or toss them into salads, leafy greens are one of nature's miracle foods. Eat them raw, or steam or stir-fry them to your liking. Just make sure to keep the heat down because they cook very quickly.

Here's why there should be a spot on your plate for leafy greens every day of the week.

Leafy green vegetables include:

- Spinach
- Kale
- Broccoli
- Red and Green Leaf and Romaine Lettuce
- Cabbage
- Edible Green Leaves: dandelion, red clover, plantain, watercress and chickweed

- Mustard greens
- Dandelion greens
- Swiss chard
- Escarole
- Turnip greens

Why Should I Eat Leafy Greens?

Disease Prevention

Leafy greens contain disease-fighting antioxidants that may help protect you from diabetes, heart disease and even various cancers. In fact, an average of 1.15 servings a day can reduce the risk of developing type 2 diabetes by 14% according to a study by the University of Leicester in England. They also are full of vitamins like zinc and vitamins A, C, and E that boost the immune system keeping your body strong. Lastly, the indole-3-carbinol found in leafy greens may prevent excess cell-division and prevent the growth of breast cancer.

Weight Loss

These vegetables have so few calories that they'll hardly even count for your daily caloric intake. Instead, you can feel free to eat them in abundance. Plus, they're packed with fiber, so they'll keep you fuller longer. Not only does fiber keep you satiated, but it also stabilizes blood sugar levels. On a diet full of leafy greens, you'll forget about those sweet cravings and sugar highs that leave you exhausted a few hours later.

Vitamin K

Greens contain high levels of vitamin K, which is essential in helping the body to properly clot blood. Vitamin K also helps slow signs of aging including bone loss, arterial calcifications, kidney damage and heart disease. A single cup of most types of leafy green vegetables will provide you with more than enough vitamin K for your *entire* day. In fact, one serving of kale provides nearly six times the recommended daily intake.

Lower Cholesterol

Dark leafy greens, particularly steamed kale and mustard greens, contain a substance called bile acid sequestrants. These sequestrants bind to bile therefore preventing the digestive system from reabsorbing them. Bile acids are typically produced by the liver and help break down fats in the gastrointestinal tract. These bile sequestrants can ultimately lower cholesterol over time because they are discarded with the roughage forcing the liver to use up even more cholesterol to produce more bile.

Eye Health

It's not only carrots that will keep your eyes sharp. Leafy green vegetables along with fruits are full of carotenoids like lutein and zeaxanthin, both of which have help improve vision biologically. You can find a wide range of carotenoids in nature, but these are the only two humans can absorb, and these are the only ones found in the visual system. They work to mitigate discomfort from glare, limit recovery times of photostress, increase your visual range, and improve your capacity to see contrast. In fact, a 2008 study suggests that the pigments might even protect the retina and prevent age-related eye diseases like cataracts and macular degeneration. If you're looking to boost your eyesight, you'll want to load up on mustard greens, Swiss chard, kale, and dandelion greens.

Vitamin B5

Escarole, a member of the chicory family closely related to endive, is packed with pantothenic acid, which is also known as vitamin B5. The B vitamins together help the body break down carbohydrates into glucose to be used as fuel on the cellular level. Unfortunately, the body cannot store excess B vitamins from day to day because they're water soluble and are excreted through urine. So, you'll need to get enough on a somewhat regular basis. What better way to boost your intake of B5 than to incorporate this lovely, dark green gem.

Calcium For Bone Health

Leafy green vegetables contain large amounts of calcium. In fact, it's the calcium that gives these foods their slightly bitter taste. While leafy greens cannot provide you with an entire day's worth of the calcium, which should range from 1,000mg-1,200mg per day, it is a great non-dairy source of this essential mineral for those who are either vegan or intolerant to lactose. To give you a general idea, a single cup of steamed boy choy provides 158g, and a serving of kale contains 139g. Though 150g won't be sufficient alone, it is an impressive amount nonetheless.

Prevent Colon Cancer

According to a BBC report, a diet rich in leafy greens and cruciferous vegetables can cut the risk of colon cancer by a stunning 46%. While these results are surely due, at least in part, to their high fiber content, scientists also believe that this effect may be thanks to the sugar galactose. Galactose helps prevents proteins like lectins from binding to the lining of the colon and causing harm.

Do you include enough leafy greens in your diet? If not, you might want to reconsider. You should, at the very minimum, eat at least 2 servings of leafy greens every single week, but more is always better!

Do You Have An Iron Deficiency?

Your body needs iron to make hemoglobin, a protein that binds to red blood cells that is responsible for carrying oxygen to the tissues. A serious, prolonged lack of iron could easily lead to a condition called anemia, a disease associated with chronic fatigue, weakness, and headaches. Though there are other ways to develop anemia, an iron deficiency is by far the most common. If you're planning to start a vegan diet, you'll want to make sure to monitor your iron levels so as to prevent the crippling effects of this disease.

Causes Of Iron Deficiency Anemia

The main causes of iron deficiency or anemia include the following:

- Blood loss. You lose blood through an injury or accident and don't have the substrates to replace the red blood cells.
- You do not absorb iron very well.
- You have heavy or frequent menstrual periods.
- You have esophageal varices, which are dilated veins in the esophagus from liver cirrhosis.
- You have gastric bleeding, which means you're losing blood from the organs that participate in digestion. Typically, this results from taking too much aspirin or other medication for arthritis.
- You have peptic ulcer disease.
- You have celiac disease, which results in malabsorption of iron.
- You have Crohn's disease, which also affects iron absorption.
- You have had gastric bypass surgery with its resultant mal-absorption syndrome.
- You take too many antacids containing calcium.
- You do not eat any meat products, and therefore have a low iron intake.
- You do not eat a diet high in iron.

Symptoms Of Iron Deficiency

If you only have a mild case of anemia, you may not have any symptoms at all, or at least not noticeable ones. When you develop symptoms, they usually come on gradually, so you might not even be aware that you're iron deficient at first. However, you'll want to keep an eye out for the following symptoms if you suspect you might be becoming anemic.

Some common symptoms of iron deficiency include the following:

- You often feel irritable
- You feel tired and weak, especially when you exercise
- You experience headaches
- You cannot think clearly or concentrate
- The whites of your eyes are bluish in color
- Your fingernails are brittle
- You develop the desire to eat things that are not food or chew on ice. (This is called pica)
- You feel lightheaded when you try to stand up
- Your skin is pale
- You are frequently short of breath
- Your tongue is sore
- You have tar-colored stools or can see blood in your stool
- You have heavy periods
- You have pain in the upper abdomen from ulcers

Diagnosis Of Iron Deficiency

The doctor will usually order a standard blood test if he suspects that you are iron deficient or suffering from anemia. He'll be looking for hemoglobin/hematocrit count, red blood cell indices, iron binding capacity or TIBC, serum ferritin, and serum iron level. If the cause of anemia is still unclear, the doctor may do a colonoscopy, an upper GI endoscopy, or a fecal occult blood test as well.

Treatment Of Iron Deficiency

If test results show that you do have iron deficiency anemia, the doctor will develop a treatment plan with you to help raise your blood levels to the point where they're considered within a normal range.

Your physician will probably suggest iron supplements to speed up the recovery process and work with you to create a regimen that will help you maintain healthy iron levels in the long-term. You can also take iron intravenously if you choose not to take the oral form.

Also, if you are pregnant or nursing, your iron requirements will be significantly higher than they would be otherwise. While breastfeeding, you'll need 6.5mg, and while pregnant, you should be getting between 22-23mg. So, you should probably be taking iron supplements anyway, but especially so if you are anemic.

It takes about two months to restore the hematocrit, the ratio of red blood cells to total blood volume, to normal. However, note that it may take up to an entire year to replenish empty iron stores completely.

Diet to Restore Iron Levels

The number one way to restore iron levels is through a healthy diet. Besides red meat, which is very high in iron, you can turn to leafy greens, fish, or even some fortified grain products. Below you'll find the foods with the highest iron content per serving.

Foods you can eat to restore your iron levels include:

- Dried Lentils
- Beans
- Peas
- Fish
- Chicken
- Turkey
- Any Kind Of Red Meat
- Peanut Butter
- Iron-fortified cereals, breads and pastas
- Soybeans
- Raisins
- Apricots
- Prunes

- Oatmeal
- Kale, Spinach And Other Types Of Greens.

Final Thoughts:

You don't necessarily have to eat a diet full of red meat to fulfill your daily iron requirements. While it can certainly help, as long as you eat a diet rich in fruits and vegetables, you shouldn't have to worry about developing anemia. That being said, we mention it here simply to warn you to stay vigilant.

B Vitamins 101

The B Vitamins are a class of water-soluble vitamins that are essential to maintaining normal physiologic and metabolic function. Included within the B-complex are eight different vitamins, namely thiamin (B1), riboflavin (B2), niacin (B3), pantothenic acid (B5), pyridoxine (B6), biotin (B7), folic acid (B9), and cobalamin (B12). Though these are all admittedly separate nutrients, they are somewhat inter-related. Mostly responsible for energy production, nervous system maintenance, and synthesis and repair of DNA and RNA, these eight vitamins are vital to human health.

Because they are water-soluble, the body cannot properly store these vitamins for later use. So, you'll need a supply of B vitamins on a fairly regular basis. A vitamin B deficiency is a very serious issue and often results in depression, memory and cognitive impairment, fatigue, nail and skin loss, and even anemia.

Vitamin B is particularly important to anyone with tinnitus because it helps to regulate the nervous system. You'll also want to pay careful attention to the amount of B vitamins you're getting if you're eating a vegetarian or vegan diet. Vitamin B comes overwhelmingly from animal sources, and those who eat a primarily plant-based diet might find themselves deficient in one of the B vitamins B12 in particular.

Below you'll find descriptions of each of the B vitamins, what their function is, and where it can be found.

Thiamin (B1)

Thiamin is a coenzyme that helps to metabolize food for energy and regulate normal heart function. Without enough thiamin, your body won't be able to convert glucose into ATP.

Surprisingly, thiamin deficiency is actually quite common in developed nations. A severe lack of thiamin can result in chronic fatigue, rapid weight loss, muscle weakness, irritability, depression, poor appetite, psychosis, nerve damage, and heart complications. The USDA recommends 1.1mg/day for women and 1.2mg/day for men, and most adults that eat a balanced diet get triple this amount on a regular basis.

Food sources include: yeasts, whole grains, beans, nuts, seeds, seaweed, liver, meat, and enriched cereals

Riboflavin (B2)

Riboflavin acts as an antioxidant preventing free radical damage. Like the other B vitamins, it supports metabolic function and promotes growth as well as skin and eye health.

Because many refined grain products are enriched with riboflavin, deficiencies are not very common in the U.S.

Symptoms of a riboflavin deficiency include thyroid dysfunction, anemia, vision problems, and migraine headaches.

Food sources include: milk, cheese, yeast, mushrooms, almonds, eggs, meat

Niacin (B3)

Niacin, also known as B3, helps maintain cardiovascular health, balance blood cholesterol levels, support brain function, and form new skin cells. It can even help regulate and prevent diabetes.

While a niacin deficiency is relatively rare in the United States, you'll recognize it by its three common symptoms when it does occur: dermatitis, diarrhea, or dementia.

Food sources include: tuna, organ meat, seeds, and mushrooms

Pantothenic Acid (B5)

More commonly known as B5, pantothenic acid is a coenzyme that is vital to metabolizing carbohydrates, proteins, fats and hormones. The energy produced by vitamin B5 helps neurotransmitters in the brain to fire. Pantothenic acid also helps in the production of red blood cells, regulation of the immune system, and creation of sex- and stress-related hormones in the adrenal gland.

Deficiencies are exceptionally unusual but are usually characterized by fatigue, depression, irritability, insomnia, vomiting, and stomach pains.

Food sources include: cheese, yogurt, asparagus, spinach, fish, eggs, chicken and fortified cereals.

Pyridoxine (B6)

Vitamin B6 helps produce hemoglobin, boost your mood, create antibodies, mitigate pain naturally, and balance blood sugar levels. It's essential to healthy nerve and metabolic function.

B6 deficiencies are relatively rare in western countries where malnourishment is uncommon. However, symptoms include irritability, anxiety, depression, confusion, muscle pains, fatigue, and even seizures in chronic cases.

Food sources include: turkey breast, grass-fed beef, avocado, pistachio nuts, tuna, pinto beans, chicken breast, sunflower seeds, sesame seeds, chickpeas

Biotin (B7)

Biotin is a coenzyme that helps to metabolize fatty acids, amino acids, and glucose. It helps give a more youthful appearance in maintaining hair, skin, and nail health. However, it usually has to be ingested orally to be absorbed properly.

Biotin deficiencies are rare, but usually are associated with dry, brittle nails, irritated skin, hair loss, muscle aches, nerve damage, cramps, and fatigue. However, you might be at risk for a biotin deficiency if you are pregnant, are using anti-seizure medication, have alcoholism, consume raw egg-whites, smoke, or have a digestive disorder.

Food sources include: liver, yeast, cheese, eggs, salmon, avocado, cauliflower, raspberries, whole grain bread.

Folic Acid (B9)

Folic acid aids in cell division and helps the body to better absorb vitamin B12, which we'll discuss shortly. The terms folic acid and folate are used interchangeably, but they are not equal. Folate is the natural source of the vitamin found predominantly in produce, where folic acid is the synthetic form commonly found in supplements. There's a discrepancy as to which is more beneficial, but both are valuable.

In 1996, the United States government mandated that companies fortify certain grain products with folic acid. This is because vitamin B9 deficiencies are very serious and can result in birth defects like spina bifida, anencephaly, and heart disorders.

Food sources include: Folate is commonly found in fruits, vegetables, and legumes. It is particularly concentrated in spinach, asparagus, avocado, black-eyed peas, brussels sprouts, romaine lettuce, and broccoli. Good sources of folic acid include beef liver and fortified rice and pasta.

Cobalamin (B12)

Vitamin B12 is important for essential brain and nervous system function and is solely obtained through animal-based products such as eggs, milk, and shellfish. Vitamin B12 is also available as a supplement at many health food shops and pharmacies.

A lack of B12 can result in serious consequences for both the brain and nervous system; at even minor levels of deficiency, symptoms such as memory loss, fatigue, and depression are common. A chronic deficiency may even result in anemia.

Food sources include: Animal foods, like beef and poultry are the only natural source of vitamin B12, along with shellfish, clams, crab, and mussels. However, many vegetarian products are fortified with B12 including, cereals, and soy-based foods.

Vitamin C 101

Vitamin C, otherwise known as ascorbic acid, is a water-soluble vitamin present naturally in many fresh fruits and vegetables.

Humans are unique insofar as they are unable to synthesize the vitamin on their own and therefore must obtain it from their diet.

The Benefits Of Vitamin C

- Vitamin C is an antioxidant that destroys cancer-causing free-radicals and helps regenerate other antioxidants
- Vitamin C helps relax blood vessels and has been shown to reduce blood pressure, LDL cholesterol, and the risk of heart disease
- Vitamin C works to lower the levels of uric acid in the blood and reduce the risk of developing gout, a type of arthritis associated with high levels of crystallized uric acid deposits in the bones
- Vitamin C helps with the absorption of iron, specifically plant-based iron, a nutrient essential to the production of red blood cells and transportation of oxygen. In fact, 100mg of vitamin C could increase iron absorption by up to 67%
- Vitamin C shortens the time required to heal wounds and strengthens the skin's natural barriers
- Vitamin C aids in the production and function of white blood cells, which fight infections

Recommended Daily Intake of Vitamin C

According to the National Food and Nutrition Board the daily recommended values for vitamin C are as follows:

- Ages 0-6 months, 40 mg per day
- Ages 7-12 months, 50 mg per day
- Ages `1-3 years, 15 mg per day
- Ages 4-8 years, 25 mg per day
- Ages 9-13 years, 45 mg per day
- Ages 14-18, 75 mg per day
- Ages 19+, 75 mg per day for women; 90mg per day for men

Best Sources of Vitamin C

The best sources of vitamin C are fruits and vegetables including citrus fruits, tomatoes, and potatoes. It can also be found in fortified grains and cereals that you might eat for breakfast. However, you will need to be careful in preparing these foods Both excessive heat and prolonged storage can destroy up to 50% of a food's vitamin C content.

Thankfully, most of these foods have a relatively short shelf-life and are generally eaten raw. Here are some of my favorite sources of vitamin C:

- Red pepper gives 158% of daily value
- Orange juice gives 155% of daily value
- One medium orange gives 117% of daily value
- Grapefruit juice gives 117% of daily value
- Kiwi fruit gives 107% of daily value
- Green pepper gives 100% of daily value
- Broccoli gives 85% of daily value
- Strawberries give 82% of daily value
- Brussels sprouts give 80% of daily value

Dietary Supplements

Dietary supplements usually take the form of ascorbic acid, which arguably has the same bioavailability as the naturally occurring alternative found in fresh fruits and vegetables.

The point has been disputed, and some research teams have found that there are differences between the naturally-occurring vitamin and the supplement. That being said, the discrepancy is not significant enough to justify any dramatic response.

Other vitamin C supplements include calcium ascorbate, sodium ascorbate, ascorbic acid with bioflavonoids, dehydroascorbate, xylonate, and threonate.

Vitamin C Deficiency

Vitamin C deficiency is a very serious condition and can result in scurvy in severe cases.

Signs of scurvy begin to show within a month without any vitamin C just as the body begins to deplete its already very limited storage. Since vitamin C is a water-soluble vitamin, any excess is usually excreted in urine.

Symptoms start out with fatigue, malaise, and other flu-like symptoms. As the disease progresses, the individual can develop gum inflammation, petechiae, purpura, and ecchymosis of the skin. It might also become increasingly difficult for the body to heal soft tissues and other wounds. Other signs of a deficiency may include swollen and bleeding gums, depression, and corkscrew hairs.

Vitamin K2: The Missing Nutrient For Heart And Bone Health

Most people have heard about vitamin K but few know that it comes in two forms: vitamin K1 and vitamin K2. Researchers have only recently discovered vitamin K2 and the crucial role it plays in bone and heart health. In fact, many claim that it is just as important as taking calcium when it comes to preventing osteoporosis and tooth decay.

Scientists have found an essential link between vitamin K2 and calcium. It turns out that without the addition of vitamin K2 either naturally or through supplementation, your body cannot properly regulate calcium levels in the blood. K2 helps to modify proteins allowing them to bind to calcium, thereby activating them. When calcium isn't absorbed and removed from the bloodstream, it ends up in the arteries instead.

Without sufficient levels of vitamin K2, you are at a greater risk of atherosclerosis and heart disease.

Unfortunately, the daily intake for vitamin K recommended by the US FDA doesn't accurately reflect the body's vitamin K2 needs. While the body can convert vitamin K1 into K2, the process is not efficient. You'll need to make sure you're eating foods that contain K2 or using a supplement to compensate.

Osteoporosis and Heart Disease

While you may assume that these two conditions have nothing to do with each other, they are actually quite closely related. The risk for both disorders increases with age, particularly in the 60's and 70's, and both conditions develop gradually over many years. In fact, atherosclerosis can begin as early as one's teens and can take years to become clinically significant enough to cause a heart attack or stroke.

Researchers at the University of California in Los Angeles have begun to study the link between atherosclerosis and osteoporosis. These disorders seem to be linked to certain regulators, namely osteocalcin and matrix GLA-protein, both of which are proteins activated by K2 for the purpose of calcium absorption. Another protein known as morphogenetic protein-2 was also shown to be relevant. It was thought to be present only in bone but has recently been found in the tissue that makes up atherosclerotic plaques.

It was found that those who suffered from osteoporosis (thinning of the bones from a loss of calcium) also had an increased risk of calcium deposits in the arteries. The reverse is also true.

What they discovered was that calcified plaques are not plaques at all but actually bone-like tissue trapped inside the arteries. That is to say that calcium deposits in the arteries can be seen as a sort of ossification of the blood vessels.

In the same way, it was found that sedentary lifestyles, diabetes, aging, smoking, and high cholesterol levels were linked to *both* osteoporosis and atherosclerosis. Scientists wondered why the conditions coexist so frequently among older adults.

Some researchers originally believed that calcium transferred itself from the bones into the arteries. However, this theory didn't hold up in clinical trials. Drugs that treat osteoporosis, such as Evista (raloxifene) and Fosamax (alendronate) work to correct the lack of calcium in the bones but do nothing to improve atherosclerosis. So, they assumed that the two disorders were regulated by separate mechanisms.

It was later discovered that vitamin K2 was the link between osteoporosis and ossification of the arteries.

Vitamin K comes as vitamin K1 and vitamin K2, the former of which is commonly found in leafy greens. Most of the research on vitamin K relates to its ability to help the liver make blood-clotting proteins, including factors II, VII, IX, and X, as well as proteins C and S. They have also found that vitamin K is a good antidote to warfarin toxicity. However, these are all qualities of vitamin K1, not K2.

More recently, it was found that vitamin K is strongly linked to the maintenance of healthy bones and the prevention of arterial plaques. Vitamin K2 seems to keep calcium out of the arteries and puts it back into the bones where it belongs.

Link Between Vitamin K2 And Osteoporosis

Osteoporosis is a huge epidemic in western countries especially among elderly women. However, those who eat foods rich in vitamin K2 significantly reduce their chance of developing the life-threatening disease. Research studies have since shown that vitamin K2 massively decreases the incidence of bone fractures. In fact, studies have shown that increased intake of K2 can reduce spinal fractures by 60%, hip fractures by 77%, and other fractures by 81%. https://www.ncbi.nlm.nih.gov/pubmed/16801507

Link Between Vitamin K2 And Heart Disease

Vitamin K2 has been found to reduce the amount of cholesterol and calcium plaques found in heart valves and in arterial walls. In one large study of more than 4800 participants, it was discovered that those who consumed more vitamin K2 reduced their risk of death as a result of heart disease by a stunning 57% because less calcium was transferred from the bones to the blood vessels.

In Conclusion

Vitamin K1 and K2 are so different in function that many have argued that they're not even the same nutrient and should be named accordingly. Hopefully, the FDA will alter the dietary recommendations to reflect daily requirements for vitamin K2 to prevent the widespread development of osteoporosis and atherosclerosis.

6 Reasons You Should Add Turmeric to Your Diet

Turmeric is a spice commonly found throughout India and Southeast Asia known for its bright yellow color and warm, piquant flavor. Originally from the curcuma longa plant, the root is ground into the powder you typically find in your supermarket.

Turmeric has been widely employed in Chinese and Indian cultures for its anti-inflammatory properties. Though the Occidental world has been slow to capitalize on the health benefits of this incredible spice, the plant's medicinal qualities have been well-documented in scientific literature in more than 10,000 peer-reviewed articles.

Turmeric's effects are most pronounced when taken as a supplement or essential oil, both of which are high in curcumin, turmeric's main active ingredient. However, you'll still derive many of the benefits simply by incorporating the spice into your weekly meals.

Anti-Inflammatory

Turmeric has long been used for its anti-inflammatory properties in Eastern cultures. Inflammation, which is at the heart of most diseases from arthritis to high cholesterol, is the body's response to infection. While inflammation is meant to help the body fight foreign invaders and repair damaged tissue, chronic inflammation can put the body's immune system into overdrive and cause major harm in the long-term.

Curcumin, the oil derived from turmeric, has even been shown to be equally as effective as typical anti-inflammatory drugs like ibuprophen and aspirin. However, there are hardly any serious side effects associated with curcumin oil. For example, turmeric helps ease pain from joint conditions, such as arthritis, where inflammation plays a key role in exacerbating chronic pain. https://www.ncbi. nlm.nih.gov/pubmed/15489888

Treatment for Inflammatory Bowel Disease

Inflammatory bowel diseases such as Crohn's disease or ulcerative colitis are debilitating disorders that affect millions of people throughout the world. However, the corticosteroids commonly given to patients only treat the symptoms and not the cause of the disease. Worse still, they damage the lining of the intestines over time actually making the condition worse. Only intended to trigger remission, these drugs do not treat the cause of the disease.

In one particular study, patients with ulcerative colitis were given curcumin oil and the drug mesalazine compared to a placebo and mesalazine were four times less likely to experience a flare up during the six-month study. Not only is curcumin oil more effective at reducing inflammation, but it actually helps support the production of healthy gut bacteria in the process. https://academic. oup.com/ibdjournal/article/15/6/935/464 7654

Indigestion and Heartburn Relief

Turmeric has also been shown to help reduce indigestion and heartburn. Typically caused by poor dietary choices, stress, alcohol, excessive caffeine, and other medical conditions, these common disorders are usually linked to inflammation.

Heart disease

High blood sugar levels and poor lifestyle choices are a major cause of oxidative stress, an imbalance between the production and accumulation of free radicals and the body's ability to detoxify itself. Oxidative stress harms the linings of the blood vessels, and cholesterol, which is used to repair the damaged areas, begins to build up inside the arteries.

Statin drugs commonly used today to treat high cholesterol levels damage the kidneys and liver, and, worse still, they only treat the symptoms and not the cause of the disorder, which is inflammation. Supplements for curcumin have actually performed better in reducing oxidative stress and inflammation than the prescription drug atorvastatin. Turmeric could prove instrumental in the war against high cholesterol, high blood pressure, heart disease, and stroke across America. https://www.ncbi.nlm.nih.gov/pubmed/18588355

Delays diabetes

Research has shown that turmeric can actually delay the onset of diabetes and help manage glucose levels in diabetic patients. Not only can it stave off type 2 diabetes, but it was found to be 400 times more effective in turning on the enzyme AMPK than metformin, a common drug prescribed for diabetes.

AMPK, seen as a therapeutic target, is instrumental in reducing insulin resistance. In fact, tetrahydrocurcumin, a fermentation made with curcumin, was actually 100,000 times more effective than metformin in activating AMPK in certain cells because of its inflammatory properties.

<u>https://www.ncbi.nlm.nih.gov/pubmed/19665995</u>

Cancer prevention

Turmeric has been shown to have important antioxidant properties, which help combat free radicals, highly reactive oxygen atoms that have been linked to cancer when at very high levels. The spice can even help the body to expel mutated cells that may have developed cancer already.

Curcumin can also help with normal liver function. The liver is responsible for detoxifying the body of xenobiotics, environmental and dietary toxins that accumulate in the body and can lead to cancer when found in excess. Because of the abnormal amounts of chemicals in the Western diet, the liver is regularly overstrained; however, curcumin can help it reclaim its normal rhythm.

Uses In Cooking

- Turmeric in dried spice form can add loads of flavor to curries, stews, stir-fries and roasted meat and chicken.
- Fresh turmeric is a root that looks much like fresh ginger. It can be juiced along with other fruits and vegetables or added to smoothies.
- It makes a great addition to a chicken marinade adding a bright orange color to the mix. In fact, turmeric is a key ingredient in Middle Eastern chicken kabobs.
- You can use turmeric as a substitute for saffron. It provides a similarly yellow hue but costs less than half what saffron does.
- Jazz up white rice by squeezing fresh turmeric through a garlic press and adding it to the rice. The turmeric offers lots of flavor, and a beautiful golden color.
- Use fresh chopped or grated turmeric in coleslaw to add color, flavor, and key nutrients.

Precautions

While some have reported allergies to turmeric when applied topically, side effects are rare and almost always mild. That being said, you should take precautions if you are on medication. Turmeric has been known to interfere with anti-coagulants such as warfarin, aspirin, and clopidogrel as well as non-steroidal anti-inflammatory drugs. You should also be very careful about adding turmeric in large doses to your diet if you are pregnant or trying to become pregnant.

You might also want to consult a medical professional if you suffer from gallbladder dysfunction, infertility, bleeding issues, iron deficiency, diabetes, GERD, endometriosis, breast cancer, uterine fibroids, or other hormonal conditions. You'll also want to avoid any supplements before a surgery as it does slow normal blood clotting. Besides these specific cases though, turmeric is a natural, harmless substance tolerated in regular doses by most people.

Chapter 12

The Different Colors in Our Plant Foods and What They Mean

IF YOU'VE NOTICED, Mother Nature has blessed us with an abundance of different-colored natural foods. The large variety of different colors of produce that we can find in nature isn't just there to make our plates look pretty. In fact, the different colors on our fruits and vegetables are generally indicative of the phytonutrients, or natural plant chemicals, that they contain. Each of these phytonutrients has special properties that can help our bodies stay healthy in many different ways. More and more nutrition experts are recommending putting a wider variety of colors on your plate to help ensure that you get a proper variety and balance of these nutrients in your body.

Here are some colorful fruits and vegetables you should consider incorporating into your diet every day for optimal health and wellness, together with the health benefits that they can bring.

Red Fruits and Vegetables

Red fruits and vegetables are typically very rich in antioxidants such as anthocyanins and lycopene. These include healthy fruits and vegetables such as tomatoes, guava, raspberries, red cabbage, watermelon, cherries, kidney beans, beets, and strawberries.

Antioxidants stop the chain reaction of oxygen-free radicals in the body that can potentially damage your cells and cellular DNA. Experts say that consuming up to thirty milligrams of lycopene can provide a great boost to health and wellness.

One medium tomato picked fresh from your garden will provide you with three milligrams of lycopene. As an added benefit, lycopene is also considered a carotenoid, which helps your body make and use vitamin A.

Orange and Yellow Fruits and Vegetables

Fruits and vegetables that come in these colors are generally rich in beta-carotene, which is a precursor to making vitamin A. Vitamin A is a healthful nutrient that helps your vision at night and also helps to control the health of your skin, bones, and teeth. These vegetables and fruits, such as yellow peppers and cantaloupes, also contain folate, which is an antioxidant that helps prevent against neural tube defects in growing fetuses.

People typically need about 500 mg of vitamin A per day, which can easily be found in just a couple of cups of yellow cantaloupe. The same amount of cantaloupe provides about 65 mg of folate, of which people generally need about 320 mg per day.

Green Vegetables

There are many green vegetables you can grow in your garden, including greens, peas, and green beans. They are especially good for the health of your bones, teeth, and eyes. You need these vegetables as adequate sources for vitamin K, which helps your blood clot better. Just two cups of raw spinach give you more than double the amount of the vitamin K you require each day for optimal health.

Green vegetables also contain great amounts of vitamin C and vitamin E, which aid in decreasing your overall risk for a wide variety of chronic diseases. Vegetables that come in this color also provide you with the phytonutrients called zeaxanthin and lutein, which protect against macular degeneration or the progressive deterioration of the part of the retina responsible for central vision that can eventually lead to blindness.

Blue and Purple Fruits and Vegetables

Blue and purple fruits and vegetables, such as blueberries and eggplant, generally contain anthocyanins, which prevent heart disease through their antioxidant properties. Fruits and vegetables that come in these colors are also known to contain certain flavonoids and ellagic acid that can destroy cancer cells, including cells that make lung cancer, pancreatic cancer, stomach cancer, and breast cancer. These compounds also have anti-inflammatory properties, which can help against colon and esophageal cancer.

White Fruits and Vegetables

White fruits and vegetables include pears, apples, cauliflower, cucumbers, and bananas. These foods are fiber-rich, which can aid in your digestion and also can bind cholesterol to prevent it from reaching the bloodstream. They contain antioxidants like quercetin, which is particularly prevalent in pears and apples. Furthermore, white fruits are known to be helpful in lowering the risk of stroke.

Chapter 13

Dealing with Existing Health Conditions You Might Have

IF YOU'RE ADOPTING a vegan lifestyle to help deal with an existing health condition or two that you might have, then you might want to look through this chapter. Here, I'll be providing tips on how to get the most out of your vegan lifestyle to help you truly beat whatever condition might be plaguing you.

Hypertension

Losing weight

As has been mentioned before, high blood pressure is linked to being overweight. Thankfully, vegan diets naturally contain lower calorie counts than diets with meat in them, meaning you should naturally lose weight, and, in turn, lower your blood pressure as well.

Avoiding salt

Consuming too much salt can contribute to elevated blood pressure levels. As such, it is best to avoid dishes that contain too much salt. If you're buying pre-prepared food, make sure to look at the label to check the sodium content. Food doesn't always have to be salty to have plenty of sodium in it, so you could already be getting more sodium than is healthy for you, even when it doesn't feel or taste like it.

Maximize the hypertension-fighting minerals in vegan foods

Many vegan foods are rich in magnesium, potassium, and other minerals that help control high blood pressure. Beans and potatoes, for instance, are great sources of these minerals. Berries contain good amounts of fiber, vitamin C, potassium, and anthocyanins, and they all work against hypertension. Whole-grain foods, such as cereals and oatmeal, also contain plenty of fiber and magnesium. Beets have been found to help lower blood pressure because of their nitrate content. In fact, according to experts, drinking a glass of beet juice can lower blood pressure in just a few hours.

Type 2 Diabetes

Monitor food intake

For vegans with type 2 diabetes, food and nutrient intake should be monitored even more closely to keep blood glucose levels within acceptable bounds. Consumption of fruits and starches should be especially moderated, and blood sugar levels should be monitored, to see how the body reacts to each specific food. Have smaller, more frequent meals.

Dividing your food intake among smaller, more frequent meals each day can help keep your blood glucose levels steady. Having meals in this way, rather than in fewer larger meals, means that the inflow of food is constant. This helps avoid spikes in blood sugar levels that the pancreas has to react to.

Chronic Kidney Disease

Cut down on sodium

The kidneys are responsible for filtering our blood. As such, diets that are high in sodium can tend to cause your kidneys to work harder than they should. Although the vegan diet can be naturally low in sodium, if you're already suffering from chronic kidney disease, taking further steps to control your sodium intake is definitely a good idea. Just like the advice dished out for hypertension above, it's really as simple as trying not to add salt to the vegan food you already have and watching the labels of the pre-prepared foods you buy for their sodium content.

Control your protein intake

As part of the body's filtration system, kidneys also have to deal with the excess protein in your body. While dumping the meat already does a lot to lower protein intake, it still pays to watch what you're eating. Have moderate amounts of plant-based foods that contain protein and try not to go overboard to give your kidneys a much-needed break.

Stay away from junk foods and processed foods

If you've already read through the rest of the book, this should be a no-brainer by now. Just to reiterate, though, many of these junk and processed foods and drinks (soda is a big culprit) contain chemicals and substances that your body doesn't want any part of, and it's your kidneys that have to pick up the slack to get rid of all of that unwanted stuff. Eat healthy foods, and your kidneys are bound to thank you for it and reward you by staying well for longer.

Constipation and Diverticular Disease

Fiber, fiber, and more fiber

Fiber simply does wonders for your digestive tract. The high-soluble fiber content from foods such as beans, lentils, whole fruits, whole grains, and vegetables helps bring more water into the colon, thus softening stools and aiding in their passage. Furthermore, studies have shown that diets high in fiber can help with the growth of friendly bacteria in the digestive tract too. Lastly, soluble fiber also helps with a more frequent passing of stool, meaning fewer amounts of bad bacteria become stuck in your digestive system, thus reducing the risk for diverticular diseases. If you're looking for foods that are high in fiber, the fruits and vegetables listed here are a good place to start:

- Carrots
- Broccoli
- Kale
- Cauliflower
- Whole apples
- Whole plums
- Whole pears
- Whole peaches
- Citrus fruits

Try to have vegetables and fruits in their natural state

Fruits and vegetables generally tend to keep more of their fiber when consumed in their whole, raw, and natural state. Cooking means you get less of the fiber content from these vegetables, while juicing does the same for fruits. So it is best to go for alternatives that keep these fruits and vegetables as close to their natural state as possible. Try having some of the foods listed above raw, and if you have a blender, consider putting your juicer away and making fruit smoothies instead, since this retains more of the fiber from the fruit's natural state.

Obesity

As has been mentioned numerous times before, a vegan diet can help a lot with weight loss, but to ensure results, other efforts must be taken as well.

Count calories

It is common knowledge that if you want to lose any weight, your body needs to burn more calories than you consume each day. Most vegans who stick to their diets will usually get no more than 1,500 calories a day, so it usually doesn't take much more than sticking to a vegan diet to see results. Still, if you want to make sure you get the results you want, try to monitor your calorie intake each day and switch out any foods with other more low-calorie alternatives.

Have smaller, more frequent meals

Breaking down your intake of food into smaller, more frequent meals means that your stomach stays at work and doesn't feel deprived, meaning you feel hungry less often too. Furthermore, it helps keep your rate of metabolism up, so that your body burns more fat and calories each day, speeding up your weight loss.

Exercise!

No healthy lifestyle is complete without proper exercise, which is especially important when you're trying to lose weight. Working out and engaging in physical activities definitely burns way more calories than just sitting around all day. So get up, get out, and be active!

Getting the right amount of exercise doesn't necessarily mean costly spending on gym memberships. Although many people go this route to great effect; exercising and being active doesn't have to cost much or lead you too far from what you'd do on a normal day. You can walk more instead of taking the bus, dance a bit when you have the time, or even just work on more household chores! There are a number of household chores that can get your heart pumping and your body burning calories, all the while you get things done around the house! Here are a few great suggestions if you're thinking about using your household chores to get more exercise.

Indoor Activities

Vacuuming. Most vacuum cleaners have quite a bit of weight in them, so when you set about vacuuming your floors, lugging that thing around can be a natural workout! Move your furniture that's been sitting in the same spots for months or years and try to get every bit of dirt in there!

Cleaning windows. Cleaning your windows is great for toning your arms, and if you've got high windows, climbing up a ladder can also serve as great aerobic exercise! Just make sure to stay safe and be careful that you don't fall over and hurt yourself, of course.

Cleaning your floors. Break out your broom and get those floors clean! Once you're done with the broom, you can also move on to a mop, or even get up close and personal with the floors for some intensive scrubbing. You'll not only get shiny floors, you'll be burning some serious calories too!

Cleaning your blinds and curtains. Many people neglect to do this as often as they should, but cleaning blinds and curtains can also burn a lot of fat. Climbing up and down a stepladder multiple times to get up to the high places for your blinds will be quite a lot of work. For curtains, the same applies, as you'll need that extra bit of height to get them down for cleaning too.

Clearing out your closets. Clearing out your closets can burn a lot more calories than it seems. Taking all that stuff and all those clothes out of the closet, transferring them somewhere you can sort them out, and putting all of the things that you want to keep back into your closet can get you burning that fat without even noticing. Not just that, you can sell off some of your unneeded stuff and earn a bit of cash in the process too!

Outdoor Activities

Mowing the lawn. If you've got a lawn, then you probably have a lawn mower too. If your lawn mower is one of those models that needs some pushing around, even better! You'll be covering quite a bit of ground just by mowing your lawn, which means you'll be burning some serious fat too!

Trimming the plants, bushes, and trees. Trimming plants outside your house can take some good hard work. You'll be dropping the pounds and ending up with a much neater-looking place as well!

Gardening. We've gone into a whole lot of detail about the benefits of starting your own home garden, so there's no way I could've missed out on adding this one! Gardening involves so many different physical activities, such as hoeing, planting, and pulling weeds, that you'll never grow bored. What's more, you can do this all summer long, making for a great long-term way to fulfil your exercise needs! The best part about it is you'll be feeding yourself with healthy plant-based food, all from your own sweat and hard work! You'll be saving money, getting the exercise you need, and eating as healthily as you can, all in one go, so it's something you should definitely try out!

Conclusion

So there you have it. The vegan lifestyle truly is a wonderful and amazing way to live. There really isn't any other way to say it—I truly, simply just love being a vegan. It has brought so much good to my life that all I can sincerely hope for, really, is that through this book, I was able to let that love shine through and share it with you.

As I mentioned, the journey through the vegan lifestyle is different for each person. No two vegans are alike, and although that may be the case, I hope that through my own journey, you've picked up a thing or two that can help you avoid the same mistakes I made and make your journey easier, more fulfilling, and more worthwhile.

That being said, this book can only take you so far. No single book in this world could ever possibly hope to impart the vast amounts of knowledge and wisdom involved in a topic as immense as veganism. Hopefully, though, you've gotten the tools you need to start learning as much as you can from your own experiences. So go out there and live your own vegan lifestyle! Try new things out, make your own mistakes (hopefully not as bad as the ones I've made), forge your own experiences and memories, share what you've gathered, and learn something new every day!

With all the love in the world, straight from the bottom of this vegan heart, thank you for taking the time to read through my humble collection of thoughts and experiences, and I wish you all the best in the many, many wonderful days ahead in your new vegan lifestyle!

Update: Within the last couple of years my pernicious anemia is no longer. According to medical professionals and all the research I have done concerning the condition it is known to be a lifelong condition. I attribute my Vegan diet for such a turnaround in my health!